The Cure & Cause of Cancer

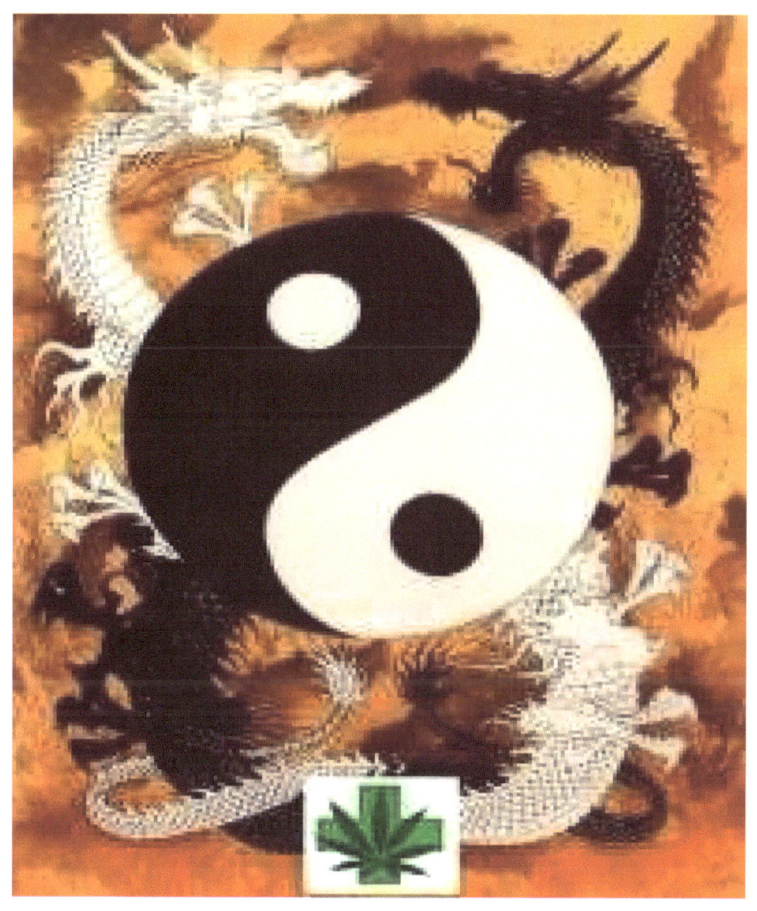

An Alternative Holistic Approach to Heal Cancer

By Ricardo B Serrano, R.Ac.

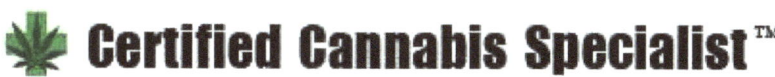

The Cure & Cause of Cancer

An Alternative Holistic Approach to Heal Cancer

By Ricardo B Serrano, R.Ac.

ISBN: 978-0-9880502-3-5

©All rights reserved.

January 30, 2013

Holisticwebs.com

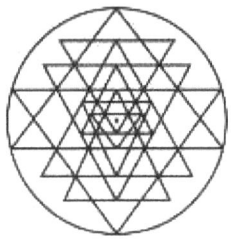

Disclaimer: The educational information in the book is for references only. Please consult your licensed physicians and not self-administer hydrazine sulfate therapy, electromagnetic healing therapy or herbs on your own. The author will not be liable for the use of the information especially in the use of diet, Hydrazine Sulfate, electromagnetic healing therapy, Guo Lin Qigong or herbs in this book.

Buenavista, Marinduque, Philippines

DEDICATION

This book is dedicated to my late dear sister Violeta Serrano Diaz who died of cancer. May the information in this book be of benefit to all patients with cancer.

"Current cannabis policies are based on fear, ignorance and greed. In reality, cannabis prohibition is a fundamental human rights violation." – Dr. Robert Melamede, PhD

"My opinion is that oral cannabis extract with equal parts THC and CBD is the ideal cancer killer without the mental effects. The cannabinoids work in concert to kill cancer; this is known as the entourage effect; THC disrupts the cancer cell mitochondria, and CBD disrupts the cell's endoplasmic reticulum, bringing certain cell death." – Biochemist Dennis Hill

"Why was cannabis made illegal? Obviously, both the pharmaceutical industry and the medical monopoly would lose billions of dollars if cannabis became the legal alternative herbal medicine (non-drug) of choice with its limitless healing potential for treating illnesses including cancer, chronic pain and depression.

Cannabis is a safe herbal medicine because cannabinoid receptor cells are lacking in the brainstem which controls breathing and heartbeat. Therefore, even strong doses do not endanger life.

Medical cannabis refers to the cured, mature female flowers of high-potency strains of cannabis.

Like "maintenance drugs" for hypertension and cholesterol, medical cannabis is meant to ease a person's suffering from debilitating health issues without the toxic side-effects of prescription drugs." – Ricardo B Serrano, R.Ac., *Certified Cannabis Specialist*

Many investigators believe that Photobiomodulation (PBM) for brain disorders will become one of the most important medical applications of light therapy in the coming years and decades. Despite the efforts of "Big Pharma", prescription drugs for psychiatric disorders are not generally regarded very highly (either by the medical profession or by the public), and many of these drugs perform little better than placebos in different trials, and moreover can also have major side-effects. – Michael R. Hamblin

The amyloid plaques in the neurons of Alzheimer's brain are removed by photobiomodulation. The Default Mode Network disruptions in the areas of the brain are also targeted and normalized. Photobiomodulation by Vielight Neuro Gamma is a non-drug effective approach that not only works for Alzheimer's but also works for: anxiety, depression, insomnia, brain injury, CTE, PTSD, stroke, autism, ADHD, Parkinson's, psychosis, addictions, attain higher meditative states and athletic performance.

Photobiomodulation by Vielight Neuro Gamma is a non-drug approach that not only works to heal depression but also works for cancer-related anxiety, insomnia, fatigue, pain, and cognitive impairment. See Photobiomodulation, pages 46, 103,111, 131, 135

As a form of Qi-healing, I personally use Vielight 655 Prime daily as an adjunct to Qigong with herbs to maintain my immune system health. I also use Vielight 810 Neuro Gamma every two days to enhance my brain function. 655 Prime or X-Plus strengthen the immune system which can be a strong deterrent to coronavirus (nCoV) infection. CBD oil, Coconut oil with X-Plus or 655 Prime intranasal light therapy (blood oxygenation), LianHua Qingwen capsules and Eight Extraordinary Meridians Qigong are the best immune system boosters to ward off viruses in my international travels. - Ricardo B Serrano, R.Ac. See page 95, Can CBD help with COVID-19 Cytokine Storm?

TABLE OF CONTENTS

Introduction 5

What is Cancer?....7 About Medical Cannabis ...17

Pot Brownie and Green Dragon Tincture............18

How Medical Cannabis Works 19

Holistic Biochemistry of Cannabinoids...................20

Spiritual and Medical Use of Cannabis...................24

Cancer and Cannabis Medicines 26

Popular Cannabis Strains 27 Before Using Cannabis 28

What causes cachexia in cancer?............................29

Hydrazine Sulfate: Unorthodox Chemotherapy....31

Tyramine-rich foods 35

Testimonials ....40 Dr. Joseph Gold speaks 41

Chanting Divine Names 45 Vagus Nerve Stimulation 46

Alkaline Ionized Water 47 True Cause of Cancer 54

Guolin New Qigong 56 Cessiac Herbal Formulas 58

Therapeutic Measures 60 How and Why Garlic Works 61

Reishi Mushroom 63 Budwig Diet for Cancer & Degenerative Diseases 70

Coconut Oil 81 Coronavirus 84 Herbs for Cancer 89 Conclusion 98

Keys to Healing 100 Electrotherapy 103 If I get cancer 104

How to Conquer Death Now 105 Cannabis and Strokes 107

Negative Ion Therapy 108 Pranic Healing 109 Get Well Verse 112

Qigong 113 Ketogenic Diet 121 Functional Medicine 122

References 126 Glossary 127 How Cannabinoids Kill Cancer Cells 132

Anti-Cancer Action 133 Final Notes 134 About the Author 135

Introduction

The information in this book "The Cure & Cause of Cancer: An Alternative Holistic Approach to Heal Cancer," was researched and written in a book format out of my desperation for answers to the wasting syndrome – cachexia – that resulted in the death of my sister from breast cancer last year. I have devoted my time during my vacation in the Philippines 2012-2013 rereading and reviewing my websites and books on cancer especially "The Cancer Industry: The Classic Expose on the Cancer Establishment by Ralph W. Moss," "Options: the Alternative Cancer Therapy Book by, Richard Walters," "Cancer's Cause, Cancer's Cure" by Morton Walker, AntiCancer: A New Way of Life by Dr. David Servan-Schreiber, MD. , Coconut Oil Miracle by Dr. Bruce Fife, ND., and Cannabis oil, Nature's Cure for Cancer by Rick Simpson.

Vital cannabis information on how cannabis works with holistic biochemistry of cannabinoids are included because medical cannabis has a great potential as a curative herbal medicine for cancer and other chronic diseases without the toxic side-effects of prescription drugs.

The excellent websites of Dr. Joseph Gold, MD, Director of the Syracuse Cancer Research Institute – http://scri.ngen.com and http://www.hydrazinesulfate.org – are full of useful information on the pathogenesis of cancer which answered the vital question "what is cancer?" "the politics of cancer," the proper use of hydrazine sulfate therapy, and why the inexpensive hydrazine sulfate was downgraded by the cancer industry's National Cancer Institute as a non-effective therapy despite its effectiveness in clinical human trials in the USA and in Russia when applied correctly - with the correct dosages and without the inclusion of alcohol, pain killers, barbiturates or tranquilizers, and tyramine-rich foods.

Basically, hydrazine sulfate inhibits gluconeogenesis (the liver's recycling of lactic acid into glucose) where the sugar is consumed in ever-increasing amounts by voracious cancer cells, and halt the leading cause of death in cancer: cachexia.

Dr. Joseph Gold said, "For the past 50 years the attention of the medical profession has been focused on the tumor. But all attempts to treat the tumor — to kill the tumor and therefore wipe out the disease — have in general been futile. During the past 50 years the death rate from this disease has reportedly hardly budged, decreasing at the most 5 percent overall, and in the major cancers not decreasing at all. Cytotoxic chemotherapy, the major weapon to defeat cancer in the last 50 years, has succeeded in killing cancer cells, but in killing normal cells, too, and has been itself a cause of cancer mortality.

Effective cancer control may lie, rather, with therapy of the 'shift' to glycolysis, than with tumor therapy, potentially obviating such developments as drug resistance and major drug toxicity. In this regard it is recognized that not only can the "metabolic shift to enhanced glycolysis" provide a basis for cancer treatment but that discovery of the regulatory mechanism(s) underlying this metabolic shift may be essential to the future development of anti-cancer therapy."

Why do I, as a licensed health care professional, recommend Hydrazine Sulfate or medical cannabis to my patients who are under the care of their medical doctors? Both hydrazine sulfate and cannabis are marketed in the United States and Canada as dietary supplements /nutraceuticals by some companies. In the United States and Canada, dietary supplements are regulated as foods, not drugs. However, I also believe that hydrazine sulfate or medical cannabis is the missing important therapeutic tool to solve the riddle of the wasting syndrome – cachexia – in cancer, and stop the voracious cancer cells to use glucose.

May the following information on cancer, *a normal body process*, the wasting syndrome that kills most patients with cancer – *cachexia* – and Hydrazine Sulfate therapy or medical cannabis benefit those people suffering from cancer.

When you get cancer, use hydrazine sulfate or cannabis as soon as possible and not wait for cachexia symptoms. The sooner you use hydrazine sulfate or cannabis, the better the results.

May the following information on alkaline ionized water, Virgin Coconut Oil rich in Medium Chain Fatty Acid (MCFA), Cessiac Yuccalive herbal formulas, Pau d'Arco, Chaparral, Guyabano, Reishi mushrooms, Dr. Beljanski's herbals, and the Budwig diet with Turmeric (Curcumin), an angiogenesis inhibitor, also be used for prevention and assist in the recovery of patients from cancer by following an integrative anti-cancer lifestyle fostering an anti-cancer terrain.

Finally, cannabis hemp oil, an angiogenesis inhibitor, and Guo Lin Qigong together with an electromagnetic healing technology invented in the Philippines can rebuild the body's Qi field by supplying negative ions needed to heal cancer and other chronic degenerative diseases.

"My studies have proved conclusively that untreated cancer victims live up to four times longer than treated individuals. If one has cancer and opts to do nothing at all, he will live longer and feel better than if he undergoes radiation, chemotherapy or surgery, other than when used in immediate life-threatening situations."— Prof Hardin B Jones. (1956 Transactions of the N.Y. Academy of Medical Sciences, vol 6)

Cancer is no longer a "death sentence" and can be cured naturally without the killing side-effects of cytotoxic chemotherapy, surgery or radiation.

Ricardo B Serrano, R.Ac., *Certified Cannabis Specialist*

Published January 30, 2013 and updated March 26, 2020, Buenavista, Marinduque, Philippines

What is Cancer? By Dr. Joseph Gold, MD, Director, Syracuse Cancer Research Institute

Cancer is said to have countless causes — a genetic cause, a cause linked to abnormal protein production, an environmental cause, and a host of other factors. In view of the fact that unlike other medical conditions such as heart disease, diabetes, stroke and others in which the death rates in the last 50 years have plummeted — as much as 70 percent — the death rate of cancer in the last half century has remained unchanged. This is in all likelihood due to our misleading conception of what cancer is. The present paper defines cancer - for the first time - as a normal body process which serves as a "protective" device to the body but which, when called upon by the body to a greater extent than possible, becomes the body's nemesis, ushering in the disease we know as cancer. While it is conceded that there are many changes associated with malignant change - genetic, mutational DNA and abnormal protein and dozens of other "components" — this paper proposes that the primary cause of cancer is not any of these changes, but energetics: that malignant change is a function primarily of energy metabolism.

Abstract. In 1931 Otto Warburg received the Nobel Prize for his demonstration that cancer cells utilize a process known as glycolysis as their chief means of energy production, rather than the more energy-efficient oxidative respiration, as in normal cells. The author later demonstrated that glycolysis acted in a two-fold manner in cancer: as a source of energy production for the tumor, as proposed by Warburg, and as a pacemaker for cancer cachexia — the weight loss and bodily debilitation causally associated with more than two-thirds of all cancer deaths. The present paper proposes that glycolysis serves a much more vital and deep-seated process to the overall integrity — and, paradoxically, downfall — of the body. In the present paper the author proposes that cancer is a normal body process, invoked as a temporary adjustment by the body to offset the development of oxidative stress - resulting from the oxygen environment and our oxygen-based metabolism and their destructive effects on tissue health, aging (senescence) and cellular and whole-body mortality.

This normal body process acts to dissipate ambient energy (ATP), necessary to the maintenance of oxidative stress, through the protective action of glycolysis and involves the body's formation of "transitional" tissues, which although morphologically normal (i.e., normal in appearance under the microscope), are metabolically "cancerous," undergoing glycolysis as their major means of energy production, but not to the extent found in cancer cells. These "transitional" tissues serve as reservoirs of glycolysis, to be activated by the body at any time and could thus 'come and go,' i.e., regress to normal body function or progress to morphologically recognizable cancer tissue. Thus when ATP availability is sufficiently decreased due to adequate glycolytic output, these tissues 'regress' to normal metabolic function.

But if ambient energy is not sufficiently lowered to offset the effects of oxidative stress, these "transitional" tissues no longer regress — their output of glycolysis is no longer "temporary" — but progress to frankly malignant tissue with maximal glycolytic activity. Once formed, however, malignant tissue— invasive and metastatic — takes on properties of its own and constitutes an imminent threat to life.

It is suggested that effective cancer control may lie with therapy of the metabolic shift to glycolysis in normal cells, rather than with therapy aimed exclusively at the tumor.

Energy Mechanics and Cancer

In 1968 I proposed that cancer cachexia was the product of a whole body energy-wasting circuit composed on the one hand of glycolysis in the 'cancer compartment' of the body and gluconeogenesis in the 'normal compartment' of the body (chiefly the liver and kidney cortex).1 Specifically it was postulated that in the anaerobic breakdown of glucose to lactic acid (glycolysis) in tumors, a net 2 ATP molecules per glucose molecule were yielded to the tumor, but synthesis of glucose, via gluconeogenesis, from the resulting lactic acid (Cori cycle2) — as well as from citrate, succinate, propionate and others — required the utilization of the equivalent of 6 ATP molecules derived from normal host sources. Thus the equivalent of at least 14 ATP was "lost" to the body economy with each specific recycling (based on 2 equivalents of "lactate" being recycled to glucose): 2 ATP molecules to the cancer cell and 12 ATP molecules from normal host tissues. This recycling process represents under abnormal or unusual circumstances a major biosynthetic pathway capable of synthesizing up to 200 grams or more of glucose per day in the adult,3,4 which exceeds total minimum daily body requirements; the only thermodynamic prerequisite for activation of this recycling process is that lactate from the glycolyzing tumor enter the blood, which multiple studies have repeatedly confirmed. 4,5

It was further specified1 that glycolysis and gluconeogenesis do not generally occur in the same tissues and were in general opposite — i.e., reverse — processes (metabolic pathways). However there were exceptions to this generality, the most important being the conversion of pyruvate to phosphoenolpyruvate (PEP). In glycolysis this conversion (PEP to pyruvate) proceeds directly, i.e., as a one-step process, catalyzed by the enzyme pyruvate kinase. In gluconeogenesis this conversion (pyruvate to PEP) is a two-step process catalyzed by the enzymes pyruvate carboxylase, which converts pyruvate to oxalacetate, and phosphoenolpyruvate carboxykinase (PEP CK), which converts oxalacetate to phosphoenolpyruvate (PEP). Thus it becomes possible to inhibit gluconeogenesis without inhibiting glycolysis, an important theoretical consideration, since many normal tissues (brain, red blood cells, skeletal muscle, others) depend on glycolysis for a portion of their energy supply. And since most gluconeogenic precursors enter the gluconeogenic pathway at the level of oxalacetate, inhibition of gluconeogenesis at phosphoenolpyruvate carboxykinse (PEP CK) is suggested as a means of inhibiting the energy loss sustained in the recycling process and therefore as a means of inhibiting cancer cachexia — associated with more than two-thirds of all cancer deaths6,7 and termed perhaps the most devastating aspect of malignancy.

In later papers it was shown that all three body substrates — carbohydrates, protein and fats — participate in this energy-wasting metabolic circuit. Protein chiefly from peripheral muscle breakdown under the influence of cancer enters the gluconeogenic pathway as amino acids at the level of oxalacetate; and fats enter this pathway as glycerol at the level of triosephosphate. All exact significant amounts of energy from normal host sources in their recycling to glucose. 8,9

Glycolysis in cancer therefore acts in a two-fold manner: as a source of energy production (growth) to the tumor and as a pacemaker for cachexia, i.e., as a source of lactate that initiates a progressive energy loss in the host through marked stimulation of gluconeogenesis. And while various substances, cytokines and others, have been proposed as the actual causative agents[10] of cancer cachexia, it should be borne in mind that no matter what the cause, cancer cachexia must proceed via a thermodynamic process.

The important consideration is that in cancer a mechanism operates to deplete the body of ambient energy.

"Transitional" Cancer

In 1966 a study was published utilizing freshly obtained human colon carcinoma and measuring the differential glycolytic rates of each cellular type within the tissue without actually destroying the original intercellular relationships and architectural integrity of the tumor mass, nor subjecting this tissue to harsh physical or chemical treatment. This was accomplished by a combination metabolic, histologic and mathematical experimental approach. [11]

This study disclosed a spectrum of glycolytic values for various tissue and cellular elements within these solid tumors, with frank carcinoma (cancer) being the highest and corresponding to previously reported values obtained by differential experimental approaches,[12,13] and normal mucosa at least 5 cm. distant from the lesion being the lowest. Specifically it was found that frank carcinoma had a glycolytic rate of 23.8 – 40.6 ul lactic acid per mg. dry weight tissue per hour, whereas normal mucosa at least 5 cm. distant from the lesion had a glycolytic rate of only 4.3 – 9.0 ul lactic acid per hour. Benign polyps, whether villous or adenomatous, had values similar to those of normal mucosa; malignant polyps, villous or adenomatous containing in situ carcinoma, were similar to those of frank cancer.

The surprising finding of this study was that the morphologically normal-appearing mucosa immediately adjacent to the invasive cancer had a glycolytic value approaching that of frank cancer — 18.75 ul lactic acid/hr — far more than that of the mucosa 5 cm. distant from the lesion. Thus, from a point of view of lactic acid elaboration (glycolysis), this microscopically normal-appearing mucosa adjacent to the lesion was metabolically almost identical to frank carcinoma, i.e., was already metabolically "cancerous." For that reason this tissue was named "transitional" mucosa (i.e., transitional carcinoma).

The presence of "transitional carcinoma" in human colon cancer was confirmed 34 years later by a team of investigators led by Isaiah Fidler,[14] using different parameters of neoplastic expression than glycolysis. Freshly obtained surgical specimens of human colon cancer were analyzed by immunochemistry for Ki-67 labeling index, epidermal growth factor receptor, transforming growth factor-a, vascular endothelial growth factor, basic fibroblast growth factor, interleukin-8, and vascular density in morphologically normal-appearing mucosa and hyperplastic mucosa adjacent to the frank, cancerous lesion, as well as in normal-appearing mucosa distant from the lesion. It was found that the expression of these factors was significantly higher in the mucosa adjacent to the lesion than in the distant mucosa and was in fact similar to their expression in the tumor itself. For this reason this adjacent tissue was given the same nomenclature as in the previously referenced study with glycolysis[11] — "transitional" mucosa. Whether this mucosa adjacent to colon cancer represented a precursor lesion or a response to the growing cancer is unclear; however, this "transitional" mucosa produced high levels of pro-angiogenic molecules, which contribute to the angiogenesis of human colon carcinoma.

Thus, from various experimental directions it has been demonstrated that, at least in human colon tissues, it is possible that morphologically normal-appearing tissue can be expressing metabolic and other biochemical characteristics of frankly malignant tissue.

Temporary or Permanent?

Can these "transitional" changes in normal tissue be temporary or must they be permanent? That is, can they 'come and go', or are they progressive, until reaching morphological identification as frank malignancy? And — need these changes occur in tissues adjacent to malignancies or can they occur in tissues de novo?

Metabolic and/or physiologic changes—"adjustments"—are common within the body. Generally these "adjustments" are temporary and act to aid the body; but if these adjustments become progressive and "permanent," they can turn markedly destructive. That is, the same devices the body calls upon that serve constructive ends, may, if allowed to progress, prove to be catastrophic.

In heat physiology, for example, as a result of exposure to high environmental heat extremes, the body calls upon — as a temporary measure — the development of a massively increased blood circulation to the skin which acts to bring needed fluid to the sweat glands, which in turn prevents or deters body heat storage by the cooling effect of evaporation of sweat; concomitantly the body develops an increased venous blood pressure, increased heart rate and increased cardiac output. But this "cooling effect" due to the massively increased skin circulation is but temporary, for if the threat of increased environmental heat energy remains undiminished — if the temporary adjustment of a massively increased skin circulation becomes permanent — the sweat glands eventually cease to function (fail) and the greatly enlarged skin circulation acts as a heat exchanger, bringing ever more ambient heat from the environment to the internal organs: to the brain, to the kidneys, to the liver; at the same time increasing venous blood pressure and cardiac output lead to high output cardiac failure. And suddenly the skin turns from cherry red to ashen grey, the cardiac output falls, and the body is plunged into heat stroke, which is very often fatal.[15,16] Thus physiological adjustments called upon as a temporary measure—especially those to an environmental threat — if allowed to become permanent, can bring on catastrophic consequences.

The question of temporary vs. permanent adjustment now calls attention to the finding of incidental cancers in the body. These are cancers that are found unexpectedly at post-mortems and by other means,[17] that have never become clinical or been diagnosed during a patient's lifetime. These clinically silent malignancies occur with surprising frequency in the prostate gland — estimated to vary between 15 percent and 70 percent with rising population age[18] — but can occur in the thyroid, breast, colon, cervix and other tissues. The findings of incidental cancer, in view of morphologically normal — appearing "transitional" cancer herein described, suggest the possibility of the existence of "transitional" cancer of different tissue types within the body, both in association with frank malignancy and de novo, which too have remained occult or undetected. While de novo "transitional" tissue may be extremely difficult to detect experimentally, a hint as to its existence — and nature — may be gained by a consideration of spontaneous regressions.

Spontaneous regressions are the occurrence of an unanticipated complete regression within the body of a clinically identifiable malignant tumor mass to its normal tissue of origin. Spontaneous regressions are extremely rare and their cause of regression is unknown. However, if there is a process within the body that can cause a frankly malignant tumor mass to undergo a complete regression to its normal tissue of origin, it is equally likely that a similar process may cause "transitional" cancer tissue — not yet morphologically malignant — to undergo regression from its newly acquired abnormal metabolic — i.e., "transitional" — functions to those functions associated with normal tissue of origin. In such a manner it would be at least theoretically possible for "transitional" tissue exhibiting metabolic aspects of cancer while morphologically normal — or disease entities themselves — to 'come and go'.

In this regard it is generally known, and confirmed in many recent studies,[19] that during early embryonic and fetal development tissues utilize glycolysis as a major pathway of energy production, and as development proceeds this pathway is in time replaced by normal oxidative respiration. Thus early embryonic and fetal tissue exemplify the same kind of energy production as found in human "transitional" mucosa — glycolytic or cancer energy production — that can regress, i.e., proceed in the direction of "normal" energy production.

But not only can metabolically 'abnormal' tissues 'lose' their abnormalities — i.e., their aberrancies disappear — the body affords examples of entire disease entities that can be "temporary," i.e. that 'come and go.' Diabetes is a classical example of this phenomenon. This disease is known to be precipitated by a number of factors, including genetic or hereditary influences, overweight, physical and psychological trauma, and many others. But this disease can also regress — disappear — totally. Examples of such regression include the diabetes of pregnancy; following the end of pregnancy this disease frequently disappears. A significant, dietary weight loss, with and without exercise, may cause this disease to fade. And for unknown reasons this disease may totally vanish.

But diabetes and the appearance of "transitional" tissues in the body have another remarkable similarity. In diabetes insulin production fails. Insulin allows glucose to get into the cells for energy production. If there is not enough insulin, glucose from the blood cannot get into the cells and instead spills out in the urine. Thus blood glucose is lost in the urine. That is, energy in the form of glucose is diverted away from the body. Like in "transitional" tissue and frankly cancerous tissues, diabetes is acting to rid the body of ambient energy.

Cancer Is a Normal Body Process

It is postulated that the diversion of energy from the body by the formation of "transitional" tissues (as well as a loss of glucose, as in diabetes), represents a metabolic adjustment which guards against the buildup of ambient energy (ATP) in the body; moreover, that the body makes this adjustment as a temporary measure, until ambient energy levels are perceived to be at "equilibrium"; at this time the "transitional" tissue returns to normal metabolic function. This process can be repeated. But if these adjustments are not temporary but are allowed to become permanent, the "transitional" tissue does not recede but goes on to become frankly, morphologically cancerous—invasive and metastatic—leading to organ dysfunction and the mortality of organ failure. While at the same time host energy loss due to increasing glycolysis and lactic acid production from functionally glycolytic ("transitional") tissues and the recycling of peripheral protein break down products and other intermediates via gluconeogenesis becomes massive, leading to cachexia—weight loss, bodily debilitation—associated with the majority of all cancer deaths. 7

Thus, it is proposed that the primary 'defect' in cancer is a normal body process that the body invokes — as a temporary adjustment — which acts to dissipate ambient energy in the body, i.e., to regulate ambient energy (ATP and ATP-equivalent) levels. This "adjustment," not only occurring in tissues adjacent to frankly malignant tumors but in tissues without such proximity, can 'come and go.' However, when this adjustment is not temporary, but becomes permanent, a panoply of changes takes place, resulting in the appearance of morphologically recognizable islands and masses of frankly malignant tissue — tumors — which take on properties of their own and become the full-blown disease entity which we today call cancer.

Of course, this hypothesis generates — as well as solves — certain problems. The prime question it generates is whether de novo "transitional" tissue can occur by itself, i.e., not in adjacency to a frankly malignant tumor mass—and then, as a one-way step, proceed and/or regress either to frank malignancy or normal tissue. The occurrence of false positive PET scans followed by negative biopsy, in the proximity of cancer and in normal tissues,20-22 presents strong evidence for this. The "false positive" indicates rapid glucose uptake (i.e., glycolysis) in the tissue under examination, but normal appearance under the microscope. While this evidence is "indirect," it is nevertheless strongly consistent with the existence of de novo "transitional" tissue.

One of the 'problems' this hypothesis solves is the question of how the presence of a relatively small amount of malignant tissue in the body — as in some cancers23 — can produce profound cancer cachexia. The answer is that the amount of "malignant" tissue is not small. There is a large component of accompanying tissue — whether "adjacent" to the lesion or not — that is in the "transitional" stage, i.e., not yet morphologically identifiable as cancer but undergoing a glycolytic — 'cancerous' — metabolism, producing copious amounts of lactic acid and stimulating host energy loss (and profound wasting) via gluconeogenesis.

The presence of "transitional" tissue can also explain another enigma—the frequency of recurrence at anastomotic sites, following a tumor resection in which the borders are declared "free" from cancer. In this instance, the borders (formerly in proximity to the resected tumor mass), although indeed "normal" in appearance under the microscope, are already metabolically malignant and serve as a forerunner to a morphologically identifiable recurrence.

More importantly, the questions must be asked: Why does the body "want" to rid itself of ambient energy? What is the threat of too much energy in the body? What function, if any, does enhanced glycolysis serve in the body?

Oxidative Stress, ATP and Telomeres

Oxidative stress is the biological stress and damage induced on living systems—enzymes, proteins, membranes, especially DNA — by reactive oxygen species (ROS), such as free radicals and peroxides, brought about by increased cellular oxidant output in the face of reduced ability of biological systems to detoxify these reactant molecules. These substances cause significant damage to tissues and organ systems, have been linked to many disease syndromes, including strokes, heart attacks and neurodegenerative disorders and can importantly affect the aging process and life span.

The production of ROS — oxidative stress — arises from oxidative phosphorylation, the initiating step of oxidative respiration, the metabolic pathway that efficiently produces relatively large amounts of ATP—ambient energy — for cellular needs (32 ATP per molecule of glucose metabolized). During oxidative phosphorylation, electron transfer results in a mitochondrial proton flow and the formation of reactant oxygen molecules. 24 Although oxidative respiration is a vital part of metabolism, ROS in the form of free radicals, peroxides and other reactive oxygen substances are elaborated. Evidence indicates that this ambient energy — ATP — may provide the energy necessary for ROS production in various living systems and be an important determinant for apoptosis (cell death). 25-27 Thus ambient energy levels are linked to oxidative stress and resulting tissue damage and dysfunction.

Telomeres are repeating DNA sequences located at the ends of chromosomes. With each cell division the telomeres become shorter. When the telomeres become too short, the cells stop dividing and cell death ensues. Telomeric length — shortening — is thus associated with senescence and the aging process as well as with cellular and whole-body mortality.

Oxidative stress — in the form of reactive oxygen species (ROS)—is well known to have deleterious consequences on telomeric length and therefore tissue function. Chronic oxidative stress, for example, compromises telomeric integrity and enhances the onset of senescence in human endothelial cells28; this same factor accelerates telomeric loss and contributes to senescence in both human cellular and in whole-body systems. 29,30

Oxidative Stress and Glycolysis

The phenomenon of glycolysis in cancer tissue has been identified as one of the fundamental questions of tumor biochemistry "not yet fully understood."31 It has been ascribed as the chief means of energy production in cancer cells (known as the Warburg effect13) and as part of a whole-body metabolic circuit important in the production of cancer cachexia.1,8 Recent evidence, moreover, indicates glycolysis might also serve another vital body function: as a protection against cellular and systemic oxidative stress. Cells in culture expressing high glycolytic rates almost totally abolish reactive oxygen species (ROS) formation.31 Pyruvate, an end-product of aerobic glycolysis, is an effective scavenger of ROS.31 Aerobic glycolysis in proliferating cells minimizes oxidative stress during the cell cycle when cell division occurs, preserving cell division and cell immortalization.32 Enhanced glycolysis renders cells resistant to oxidative stress, modulating cellular and organism senescence with significant increases in life span. 31-33

Cancer, Senescence and Immortality

This paper presents — in particular, the body's evolution of glycolysis and functionally glycolytic ("transitional") tissue — essentially as a normal process which the body invokes as a protective device to offset the destructive effects of the oxygen environment in which we live. Oxidative stress — an inevitability of our oxygen-based metabolism — exerts markedly injurious effects on tissue and organ systems, on aging and on mortality itself. In the form of reactive oxygen species (ROS), oxidative stress and its damaging effects extend to all tissues, particularly to the telomeres and cell division, with important consequences on senescence and life span. But oxidative stress seems to be at least partially dependent on ambient energy — ATP — to fuel ROS production. And in lessening ambient energy levels, among other mechanisms, 31-33 glycolysis acts to counter the availability of these cell-damaging molecules.

Glycolysis by itself, instead of making available 32 ATP per glucose molecule for general cellular needs by oxidative respiration, produces only 2. And in conjunction with gluconeogenesis — and the nearly obligatory recycling of tumor-produced lactate to glucose — glycolysis removes 14 ATP from the general body economy with each glucose molecule metabolized (2 ATP to the glycolyzing tissue, 12 ATP from normal body energy pools). The loss of ATP to the body economy as a consequence, can become considerable. Thus, in making less ATP available for elaboration of ROS, glycolysis functions as an effective inhibitor of oxygen stress in the body.

To what extent can glycolysis be invoked by the body as a defense against oxidative stress? Other than frank cancer tissue, the body — seemingly — has but one choice: the elaboration of "transitional" tissue. As discussed, these are tissues in proximity to a cancerous lesion that appear normal morphologically but are already metabolically "cancerous," undergoing glycolysis as their major means of energy production, as well as expressing other metabolic and biochemical characteristics of frankly malignant tissue. Are these "transitional" tissues real?

The two previously referenced studies[11,14] indicate the affirmative. These two studies, one completed 34 years after the other, using the same investigational tissue — freshly obtained human colon tumor tissue — and employing totally unlike experimental procedures, found almost identical results: namely, that the morphologically normal-appearing tissue adjacent — i.e., in close proximity — to the cancerous lesion, metabolically more closely resembled the cancerous lesion than the same normal-appearing tissue distant from the lesion. Each study independently named this adjacent tissue "transitional." That these almost identical results could be a random "coincidence" is only a remote possibility.

Does de novo "transitional" tissue exist? That is, not in association with any cancerous lesion? This is an important question, for if so, such tissue could serve as reservoirs of glycolysis and be activated by the body at any time. Previous evidence for the existence of de novo "transitional" tissue in the body has been set forth — principally in the form of false positive PET scans followed by negative biopsy — indicating rapid glycolysis (F18 2-deoxyglucose uptake) in the tissue examined, but normal appearance under the microscope. Although false positives occur in tissues exhibiting hyperplasia, granulomas and in other inflammatory conditions, false positive PET scans in the proximity of cancer and in normal tissues — which can be high in incidence[21] — constitute strong presumptive evidence of the presence of de novo "transitional" tissue in the body; and, thus, that this tissue can 'come and go.'

But to answer this question more particularly, the transition between a morphologically normal and a morphologically malignant cell must be considered. Does a normal cell become cancerous in one step? That is, at one moment is it totally normal and the next, totally malignant? The findings presented in this paper, namely, that it is possible that morphologically normal-appearing tissue under the microscope can be expressing metabolic characteristics of frankly malignant tissue, suggests that the likelihood is greater that a normal cell reaches malignancy through intermediate stages rather than "turns" malignant at once.

But, if so, such intermediate stages constitute de novo "transitional" tissue — which would seemingly be applicable to many, if not all, cancers. Thus the probability is high that de novo "transitional" tissue plays a key role — actually is a sine qua non — to the development of definitive cancer.

Moreover, if increased glycolysis via the development of "transitional" tissues represents a normal process invoked by the body as a temporary adjustment, which acts to regulate ambient energy levels in restraint of oxidative stress, the implication, as previously discussed, is that these tissues 'come and go.' Thus when ATP availability is sufficiently decreased, these tissues "regress" to normal metabolic function.

But if ambient energy is not sufficiently lowered to offset the effects of oxidative stress, these "transitional" tissues no longer regress — their output of glycolysis is no longer "temporary" — but go on to form tissues with maximal glycolytic capacity, i.e., frankly, morphologically identifiable malignant tissue. Once formed, however, malignant tissue, invasive and metastatic, takes on properties of its own and constitutes an imminent threat to life.

Since this paper identifies a "normal body process" — the shift to glycolysis in normal tissues — to be the primary "defect" in cancer and this shift's "aberration" to result in tumor formation, the question arises as to which aspect of tumorigenesis may provide a potentially more effective basis for cancer therapy: the metabolic 'shift' or the tumor?

For the past 50 years the attention of the medical profession has been focused on the tumor. But all attempts to treat the tumor — to kill the tumor and therefore wipe out the disease — have in general been futile. During the past 50 years the death rate from this disease has reportedly hardly budged, decreasing at the most 5 percent overall, and in the major cancers not decreasing at all.34 Cytotoxic chemotherapy, the major weapon to defeat cancer in the last 50 years, has succeeded in killing cancer cells, but in killing normal cells, too, and has been itself a cause of cancer mortality.

Effective cancer control may lie, rather, with therapy of the 'shift' to glycolysis, than with tumor therapy, potentially obviating such developments as drug resistance and major drug toxicity. In this regard it is recognized that not only can the "metabolic shift to enhanced glycolysis" provide a basis for cancer treatment but that discovery of the regulatory mechanism(s) underlying this metabolic shift may be essential to the future development of anti-cancer therapy. 33

It is here theorized that cancer is a normal process invoked by the body as a protective device against tissue damage, senescence and death. It is the most exquisite of paradoxes that the more the body calls upon glycolysis to combat oxidative stress, the more likely it is that the body's protective mechanism will lead to its almost certain confrontation with death.

References

1. Gold, J. Proposed treatment of cancer by inhibition of gluconeogenesis. Oncology 22: 185-207, 1968.
2. Cori, C. F. Mammalian carbohydrate metabolism. Physiol. Rev. 11: 143-275, 1931.
3. Krebs, H. The Croonian Lecture, 1963. Gluconeogenesis. Proc. Roy. Soc. (London) Ser. B 159: 545-564, 1964.
4. Reichard, G. A. et al. Quantitative estimation of the Cori cycle in the human. J. Biol. Chem. 238: 495-501, 1963.
5. Demartini, F. E. et al. Lactic acid metabolism in hypertensive patients. Science 148: 1482-1483, 1965.
6. Robins, S. Textbook of Pathology (W.B. Saunders, Philadelphia), 1957.
7. Brauer, M. et el. Insulin protects against hepatic bioenergetic deterioration by cancer cachexia. An in vivo 31P magnetic resonance study. Cancer Res. 54: 6383-6386, 1994.
8. Gold, J. Cancer cachexia and gluconeogenesis. Ann. N.Y. Acad. Sci. 230:103-119, 1974.
9. Gold, J. Hydrazine sulfate: A current perspective. Nutrition and Cancer 9: 59-66, 1987.
10. Ohnuma, T. in Cancer Medicine (eds. Kufe, D.W., Pollock, R.E. Weichselbaum, R.R et al. (B. C. Decker, 2004), pp. 2427-2428.
11. Gold, J. Metabolic profiles in human solid tumors: I. A new technic for the utilization of human solid tumors in cancer research and its application to the anaerobic glycolysis of isologous benign and malignant colon tissues. Cancer Res. 26: 695-705, 1966.

12. Kidd, J., Winzler, R. J. & Burk, D. Comparative glycolytic and respiratory metabolism of homologous normal, benign, and malignant rabbit tissues, with particular reference to the benign virus papilloma (Shope) and a transplanted cancer derived therefrom (the V2 carcinoma). Cancer Res. 4: 547-553, 1944.
13. Warburg, O. On the origin of cancer cells. Science 123: 309-314, 1956.
14. Kuniyasu, H., Wataru Y., Shinohara H., Yano S., Ellis L.M., Wilson M.R., Bucana C.D., Rikita T., Tahara E. & Fidler, I.J. Induction of angiogenesis by hyperplastic colonic mucosa adjacent to colon cancer. Am. J. Pathol. 157: 1523-1535, 2000.
15. Gold, J. Development of heat pyrexia. J. Am. Med. Assoc. 173: 1175-1183, 1960.
16. Gold, J. in Medical Climatology (ed. Licht, S.) Ch 14 (E. Licht, New Haven), 1964.
17. Zhuang, H. et al. Incidental detection of colon cancer by FDG positron emission tomography in patients examined for pulmonary nodules. Clin. Nuclear Med. 27: 626-632, 2002.
18. Gittes, R. F. Carcinoma of the prostate. N. Engl. J. Med. 324: 236-245, 1991.
19. Dumollard, R. et el. Mitochondrial function and redox state in mammalian embryos. Semin. Cell Dev. Biol. 20: 346-353 (2009).
20. Moscowitz, C. H., Schuder, H., Teruga-Feldstein, J. et al. FED-PET in Advanced-Stage Diffuse Large B-Cell Lymphoma. J. Clin. Oncol. 28: 1896-1903, 2010.
21. Asad, S, Aquino S. L., Ptyavisetput, V. and Fischman, A. J. False Positive FDG Positron Emission Tomography Uptake in Nonmalignant Chest Abnormalities. Am. J. Roentgenology 182: 983-989, 2004.
22. Schrevens, L., Lorrent, N., Dooms, C. and Kansteenkiste, J. The Role of PET Scans in Diagnosis, Staging, and Management of Non-Small Cell Lung Cancer. The Oncologist 9: 633-643, 2004
23. Nathanson, L. & Hall, T. C. A spectrum of tumors that produce paraneoplastic syndromes. Ann. N.Y. Acad. Sci. 230, 367-377, 1974.
24. Schultz, B. & Chan, S. Structures and proton pumping strategies of mitochondrial respiratory enzymes. Annu. Rev. Biophys. Biomol. Struct. 30: 23-65, 2001.
25. Cruz, C. M., Rinna , A., Forman, H. J., Ventura, A. L., Persechini, P. M. & Ojcius, D. M. ATP activates a reactive oxygen species-dependent oxidative stress response and secretion of proinflammatory cytokines.in macrophages. J. Biol. Chem. 282: 2871-2879, 2007.
26. Bhatnagar, A. Contribution of ATP to oxidative stress-induced changes in action potential of isolated cardiac myocytes. Am. J. Physiol., Heart and Circulatory Physiology 272: 1598-H1608, 1997.
27. Richter, C., Schweizer, M. Cossarizza, A. & Franceschi, C. Control of Apoptosis by the cellular ATP level. FEBS Letters 378: 107-110, 1996.
28. Kurz, D.J., Decary, Y.H., Trivier, E. Akhmedov, A. and Erusalimsky, J.D. Chronic oxidative stress compromises telomere integrity and accelerates the onset of senescence in human endothelial cells. J. Cell Sci. 117: 2417-2426, 2004.
29. Tchirkov, A & Lansdorp, P.M. Role of oxidative stress in telomere shortening in cultured fibroblasts from normal individuals and patients with ataxia-telangiectasia. Human Mol. Genetics 12: 227-232, 2003.
30. von Zglinicki, T. Oxidative stress shortens telomere. Trends Biochem. Sci. 27: 339-344, 2002.
31. Brand, K. Aerobic glycolysis by proliferating cells: Protection against oxidative stress at the expense of energy yield. J. Bioenergetics Biomembranes 29: 355-364, 1997.
32. Kondoh, H., Lieonart, M.E., Bernard, D. & Gil, J. Protection from oxidative stress by enhanced glycolysis; a possible mechanism of cellular immortalization. Histol. Histopathol. 22: 85-90, 2007.
33. Kondoh, H. Cellular life span and the Warburg effect. Exp. Cell. Res. 314:1923-1928, 2008.
34. Kolata, G. As other death rates fall, cancer's scarcely moves, The New York Times, April 24, 2009.

About Medical Cannabis

Medical cannabis refers to the cured, mature female flowers of high-potency strains of cannabis.

Inhaled cannabis: smoked, vaporized, converted

- Bud: the dried, manicured, mature female cannabis flower
- Sinsemilla: seedless cannabis bud
- Kef: powdery resin glands (trichome)
- Hashish: compressed resin glands
- Oil: (Hash or grass) liquefied resin glands

Eaten: oral ingestion (WARNING: Eaten cannabis takes up to an hour to take effect. Avoid overdose by waiting to use more.) All the various forms listed above can be heated and eaten

- Butter: used for cooking edibles
- Tincture: ethyl alcohol (liquor)-based by the dropper
- Food: pastries, brownies, candies, sauce using any of the above
- Mari-pills: encapsulated cannabis in oil

Topical use: external, transdermal application:

- Salve: cream or oil-based compounds or suspensions
- Tincture: ethyl alcohol (liquor)-based suspensions
- Liniment: isopropyl (rubbing) alcohol-based or DMSO-based suspensions

Important Facts on medical cannabis:

- The bud portion of the plant has a coating of resin glands that contain cannabinoids, the active compounds. The cannabinoids attach to special receptor sites in the brain and other parts of the body.
- In general, cannabis is used to treat symptoms rather than cure disease. Smoked cannabis provides rapid and efficient delivery. Since many health problems cause similar symptoms, people with a variety of diseases all benefit at a basic level: Relief from physical or mental suffering.
- Cannabis is non-toxic, however, as with any other medication, one should always begin by using a low dosage and increase it as needed.
- Cannabis brings relief to a wide variety of body systems and ills. Cannabis resin and its derivatives have long been used to treat symptoms of many health conditions. Among these maladies are:

ADD / ADHD, AIDS, anorexia, anxiety, heart disease, arthritis, asthma, ataxia, bipolar, cachexia, cancer, chronic fatigue, chronic pain, cramps, Crohn's, depression, epilepsy, fever, glaucoma (progressive blindness), HIV, insomnia, migraine, MS, nausea, neuralgia, neuropathy, PMS, PTSD, rheumatism, sickle cell anemia, spasms, spinal injury, stress, vomiting, wasting syndrome, tinnitus, Alzheimer's, senility, lowers blood pressure.

How does one know where to start? First look at what specific symptoms need to be treated, then see if there are any negative effects that contraindicate its use. That will help a patient to identify the appropriate form, dosage and means of ingestion. Cannabis is exceptionally safe, physically. Not one single death due to cannabis overdose has been reported in medical history.

Reference: Cannabis Yields and Dosage by Chris Conrad, 2010

The World's Best Pot Brownie Recipe

Pot brownie recipe for an 8 x 8-inch brownie pan:

- 1/2 ounce cannabis
- 1/2 cup vegetable oil
- 1/4 teaspoon baking powder
- 1/4 teaspoon salt
- 1/2 cup flour
- 1/3 cup cocoa powder
- 1 cup sugar
- 2 eggs
- 1 teaspoon vanilla

Grind the cannabis in a coffee grinder or equivalent until it has the consistency of coarse dust. Spread evenly onto a frying pan, preferably nonstick. Use the smallest pan possible and the largest burner available to ensure that the entire surface is evenly heated. Add the vegetable oil, preferably coconut oil. Turn on heat to medium until oil begins to smoke, then turn down to the lowest possible setting. Let the oil/cannabis mixture simmer for at least an hour, stirring frequently. Remove from heat and strain the oil through a coffee filter.

Mix the dry ingredients in one bowl. In a second, larger bowl, mix the cannabis-infused oil and sugar (preferably honey), then add eggs and vanilla. When blended, add the dry ingredients. Pour into a greased 8 x 8-inch pan and bake for 20 minutes at 350 degrees.

Green Dragon Tincture

Start with a couple of buds. Then take a pure form of ethanol, like vodka or grain alcohol. Throw the buds in, and let them sit for a couple of weeks. Then you simply strain through a sieve and enjoy what is known as green dragon tincture.

The green dragon tincture and pot brownie recipes will deliver THC and CBD in amounts that are large enough to have an effect which is similar to smoking or vaporizing cannabis. Commercial cannabis-infused ointment (salve) can be also used topically for topical pain relief.

Reference: Stoned by Dave Casarett, MD, 2015, pages 98 - 99 and 261

References on Cannabis and Endocannabinoid system:

- How Cannabis Works, page 19; Holistic Biochemistry of Cannabinoids, page 20
- Spiritual and Medical Use of Cannabis, page 24 - 25
- Cancer and Cannabis Medicines, page 26; Popular Cannabis Strains, page 27
- Before Using Cannabis, page 28; Cannabis Hemp Oil, page 96
- Endocannabinoid system, Conclusion, page 98
- Cannabis and Strokes, page 107
- Endocannabinoid Deficiency, page 112
- Cannabis, acupuncture and Qigong, page 113
- Treating depression, chronic pain and anxiety disorders with medical cannabis, page 131
- How Cannabinoids Kill Cancer Cells, page 132
- Cannabis hemp oil is antiangiogenic, page 134

How Cannabis Works

Endocannabinoids (Brain Derived)
Foods: Omega-3s & Omega-6s
Anandamide (AEA)

Phytocannabinoids (Plant Derived)
Buds, Tinctures, Extracts
THC, CBD, CBN, etc.

Synthetic Cannabinoids (Pharmaceutical Lab)
Patented Synthesized Compound
THC-only (Marinol)

↓

Endocannabinoid Receptors (Brain Receptors)

CB1, CB2, etc.

The endocannabinoid system (ECS) is involved in regulating a variety of physiological processes including appetite, pain and pleasure sensation, immune system, mood, and memory.

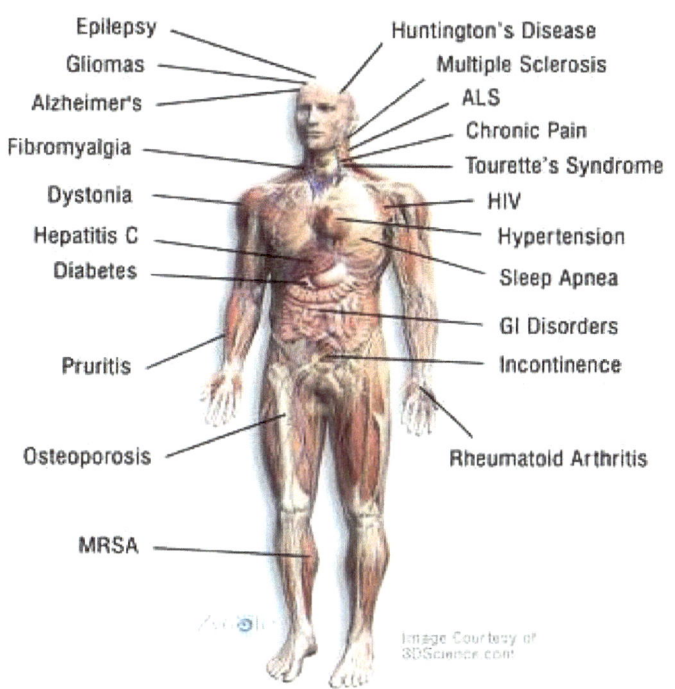

- Epilepsy
- Gliomas
- Alzheimer's
- Fibromyalgia
- Dystonia
- Hepatitis C
- Diabetes
- Pruritis
- Osteoporosis
- MRSA
- Huntington's Disease
- Multiple Sclerosis
- ALS
- Chronic Pain
- Tourette's Syndrome
- HIV
- Hypertension
- Sleep Apnea
- GI Disorders
- Incontinence
- Rheumatoid Arthritis

Potential Therapeutic Uses of Medical Marijuana

"So many lives could have been saved if only you had believed in me sooner." - Cannabis

Holistic Biochemistry of Cannabinoids by Dr. Robert Melamede, PhD

The following quotations from Dr Melamede's video show that cannabis is an important herb that supplies important essential nutrients (phytocannabinoids) to the body's endocannabinoid system essential for health maintenance and therapy especially for cancer and other diseases. Dr. Robert Melamede, a biology biochemist, believes that the endocannabinoid system could be responsible for the regulation and balance of the body's essential processes and systems.

"Endocannabinoids are the oil of life. And what they do is minimize. It's friction we're talking about. Biochemical friction essentially and what we'd like to do is minimize the consequences, essentially, we don't want ourselves wearing out. So we need to oil ourselves appropriately, and our bodies try to do that, but there is a direction to our imbalance because even though we're all unique and we're all different, we all share a certain characteristic. We're all getting older and that age is attributable to the accumulated damages that are occurring from that friction and we'll elaborate on that a little more because as was pointed out by Dr Mephlam, these things have constructive roles as well, they are part of signalling mechanisms.

So free radicals act as chemical messengers they allow us to realize there is an imbalance, and when I say us, I mean at a chemical level between ourselves, between our organs and between us as individuals, formations in our societies, how we fix things.

But certainly on a chemical level, free radicals tell us that something is wrong, let's try to fix it. But alternatively they say something's wrong, let's kill it, because we don't want, for example, genetically damaged cells in us. If we can't fix those genetically damaged cells, then we have mechanisms to do that – DNA repair mechanisms – then we get rid of those cells because these are the cells that go on to become cancer.

Is marijuana the ultimate holistic medicine if it is coordinating and balancing all of these different organised entities within our body. Or is it the devil's weed as others would have us believe?

So we are seeing it working on a sub cellular level. We see that leading up to consciousness demean by transcending scales and how its effect on consciousness has an impact on society. This is why cannabinoids have such a unique evolutionary role because they are transcending like this. So cannabinoids regulate cardiovascular health and this is all work sponsored by the NIH and researchers all around the world. This is coming out of peer reviewed journals. I don't talk about my research since I became chairman of the biology department. That's when I shifted to cannabinoid research and it goes very very slowly when you have to waste all your time being chairman.

So cannabinoids regulate cardiovascular health and what you see here is when you have a heart attack blocking oxygen and eventually the oxygen re flows and you have a ischemia reperfusion that generates injury. That injury is free radical associated. Here what you see is that you reduce the cell death in your heart through the endocannabinoid system, so presumably exocannabinoids of various forms will have similar effects.

..Dealing with the heart, with arrhythmia and cell death, and in both cases, the cannabinoids prevent cell death and prevent arrhythmia which are fundamental problems when you have cardiovascular disease.

..It's regulating the digestion system, so we see that the pharmacological modulation of the endocannabinoid system can provide new therapeutics for a number of diseases. Things like gastro intestinal disease, paralytic ileus, Crohn's disease, irritable bowel syndrome and a whole variety of digestive system related illnesses where people who are using cannabinoids know it works. This is the foundation for it. It's this balancing act again of trying to restore biochemical health, essentially.

Cannabinoids have a profound effect on the nervous system. The key component here of this is even if these studies aren't as positive as many expect them to be, that we are only just beginning to appreciate the huge therapeutic potential of this family of compounds is clear.

For multiple sclerosis, for pain, for spasticity, for a whole variety of neurologically related imbalances, the endocannabinoid system is how your body is trying to fix you, and if you're not being fixed, that means you need more, so the ideal medicine is often not the little purple pill that you see on TV or any of the variety of things. In my mind, the first choice medicine should be cannabinoids when there is an indication for it because they are mimicking what your body is doing."

Source: Excerpts from video Holistic Biochemistry of Cannabinoids, January 20, 2014

References on Cannabis and Endocannabinoid system:

- Spiritual and Medical Use of Cannabis, page 24
- Cannabis Hemp Oil, page 96
- Endocannabinoid system, Conclusion, page 98
- Cannabis and Strokes, page 107
- Endocannabinoid Deficiency, page 112
- Cannabis, acupuncture and Qigong, page 113
- Treating depression, chronic pain and anxiety disorders with medical cannabis, page 131
- How Cannabinoids Kill Cancer Cells, page 132
- Cannabis hemp oil is antiangiogenic, page 134

Active Ingredients: (Cannabinoids)

There are approximately 60 identified cannabinoids and each of an infinite number of strains of cannabis has its own cannabinoid profile.

The active cannabinoids each have unique physiological effects and many combinations actually appear to have synergistic and antagonistic effects.

Delta-9-tetrahydrocannabinol (THC):

Euphoric, stimulant, muscle relaxant, anti-cancer, anti-epileptic, anti-emetic, anti-inflammatory, appetite stimulating, bronchio-dilating, hypotensive, anti-depressant and analgesic effects.

Study finds THC promotes death of brain cancer cells and shrinks tumors *

Tetrahydrocannabivarin (THCV, THV), also known as **tetrahydrocannabivarol**:

A non-psychoactive cannabinoid found naturally in Cannabis sativa. It is an analogue of tetrahydrocannabinol (THC) with the sidechain shortened by two CH2 groups. THCV can be used as a marker compound to differentiate between the consumption of hemp products and synthetic THC (e.g., Marinol). THCV is found in largest quantities in Cannabis sativa subsp. sativa strains. Some varieties that produce propyl cannabinoids in significant amounts, over five percent of total cannabinoids, have been found in plants from South Africa, Nigeria, Afghanistan, India, Pakistan and Nepal with THCV as high as 53.69% of total cannabinoids. They usually have moderate to high levels of both THC and Cannabidiol (CBD) and hence have a complex cannabinoid chemistry representing some of the world's most exotic cannabis varieties. It has been shown to be a CB1 receptor antagonist, i.e. blocks the effects of THC. In 2007 GW Pharmaceuticals announced that THCV is safe in humans in a clinical trial and it will continue to develop THCV as a potential cannabinoid treatment for type 2 diabetes and related metabolic disorders, similar to the CB1 receptor antagonist rimonabant.

Cannabidiol (CBD):

A major constituent of medical cannabis. CBD represents up to 40% of extracts of the medical cannabis plant. Cannabidiol relieves convulsion, inflammation, anxiety, nausea, and inhibits cancer cell growth. Recent studies have shown cannabidiol to be as effective as atypical antipsychotics in treating schizophrenia. In November 2007 it was reported that CBD reduces growth of aggressive human breast cancer cells in vitro and reduces their invasiveness. It thus represents the first non-toxic exogenous agent that can lead to down-regulation of tumor aggressiveness. It is also a neuroprotective antioxidant. Also lessens the psychoactive effects of THC and has sedative and analgesic effects.

Cannabichromene(CBC): Promotes the effects of THC and has sedative and analgesic effects.

Cannabigerol (CBG): Has sedative effects and anti-microbial properties as well as lowering intra-ocular pressure. CBG is the biogenetic precursor of all other cannabinoids.

Cannabinol (CBN): A mildly psychoactive degradation of THC, it's primary effects are as an anti-epileptic, and to lower intra-ocular pressure.

There are many strains of high quality cannabis from 100% Sativa and 100% Indica to Sativa-Indica hybrid crosses, an alternative to using Heavy Narcotic Pharmaceuticals like Oxycontin or Morphine, and other antidepressant drugs such as Valium and Benzos.

Cannabis can be taken by: 1. vaporizing (rather than smoking); 2. eating; and 3. Topically.

See Pot Brownie Recipe and Green Dragon Tincture, page 18; Cannabis and Strokes, page 107; Treating depression, chronic pain and anxiety disorders with medical cannabis, page 131; How Cannabinoids Kill Cancer Cells, page 132

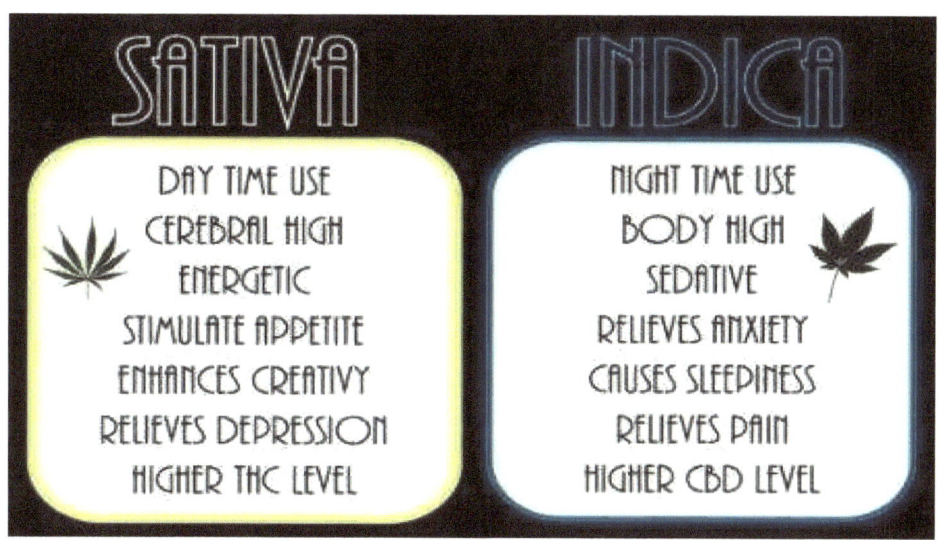

Cannabis Sativa and Indica Strains

What conditions can be treated with cannabis?

- ADHD
- AIDS/HIV
- Anxiety/Stress Disorder
- Arthritis
- Asthma
- Brain/Head Injury
- Cancer
- Cerebral Palsy
- Chemotherapy Treatment
- Chronic Pain
- Colitis
- Crohn's Disease
- Depression
- Eating Disorders
- Eczema
- Emphysema
- End of life/Palliative care
- Epilepsy

Fibromyalgia
Glaucoma
Hepatitis C
Irritable Bowel Syndrome
Chronic Migraines
Multiple Sclerosis
Muscular Dystrophy
Nausea – Chronic and debilitating Neuralgia
Paraplegia/Quadriplegia
Psoriasis
Parkinson's Disease
Radiation Therapy
Seizure Disorders
Sleep Disorders
Spinal Cord Injury
Substance Addiction/Withdrawal

Properties and Uses: Although the current interest in cannabis centers on its euphorigenic properties, the plant has in the past also shown much promise as a medicinal agent. One researcher's catalog of past uses includes: analgesic-hypnotic, topical anesthetic, antiasthmatic, antibiotic, antiepileptic and antispasmodic, antidepressant and tranquilizer, antitussive, appetite stimulant, oxytocic, preventive and anodyne for neuralgia (including migraine), aid to psychotherapy, and agent to ease withdrawal from alcohol and opiates. - The Herb Book by John Lust, 1974, page 146.

Spiritual and Medical Use of Cannabis

Spiritual well-being is widely accepted as an important part of overall health. Spiritual use of cannabis relates to seeking a sense of meaning, enlightenment and connection.

Cannabis has a rich history of spiritual use. It is listed as one of the five holy plants in the Atharvaveda, a sacred Indian text from the second millennium BCE. The Scythians, who lived in what is now Eastern Europe, used cannabis at funerals to pay respect to departed leaders. Ancient Chinese texts say that cannabis can lighten a person's body and allow them to communicate with spirits. The Persian prophet Zoroaster (7 BCE) relied on the intoxicating effects of bhanga, a cannabis drink, to bridge heaven and earth. Some researchers believe that kannabosm, a plant mentioned in the Old Testament as an ingredient in the sacred anointing oil, was an ancient name for cannabis.

Today, some people use cannabis in their spiritual practice. Rastafarians and some Hindus and Sikhs use cannabis in religious ceremonies. Other people use it in ways they consider spiritual, such as for reflection, contemplation or personal growth. The relaxing effects of cannabis help some people gain a different perspective when trying to understand difficult life situations. Some believe that cannabis, as a plant, has something to teach them.

Cannabis is used by some to increase an appreciation for and connection with nature. People also use cannabis to bond with each other. These feelings of connectedness contribute to an overall sense of "oneness."

"Marijuana actually, what it does to me beyond all other social aspects of it, it actually really combines me with nature. A lot of my religious experiences have actually come through marijuana. It is just that connection, an awareness of yourself, I think, and that you are part of nature…" "When you ingest plants that have psychoactive effects, it's sort of like the consciousness of the plant expresses itself vicariously through your body and your mind… I like to use it for learning and to gain knowledge on how to treat people and how to live…"

Medical Use of Cannabis

However, about 4% of Canadians (1.2 million people) use cannabis medicinally. In BC, about 200,000 people report using cannabis as medicine. Cannabis is used to treat many medical conditions and symptoms. It is effective in treating nausea, loss of appetite, pain, anxiety, insomnia, inflammation and muscle spasms. These symptoms are often part of physical or mental conditions. Arthritis, cancer, HIV/AIDS, multiple sclerosis, epilepsy, Parkinson's disease, ADHD and post-traumatic stress disorder are some conditions cannabis can help treat.

Sometimes cannabis is more effective than pharmaceutical drugs and has fewer negative side effects. Some people use cannabis to help them cope with the side effects of, or to replace, these medications. Others use cannabis to deal with withdrawal symptoms from other legal or illegal drugs.

Source: **Why people use cannabis** by **Rielle Capler** http://www.heretohelp.bc.ca/visions/cannabis-vol5/why-people-use-cannabis

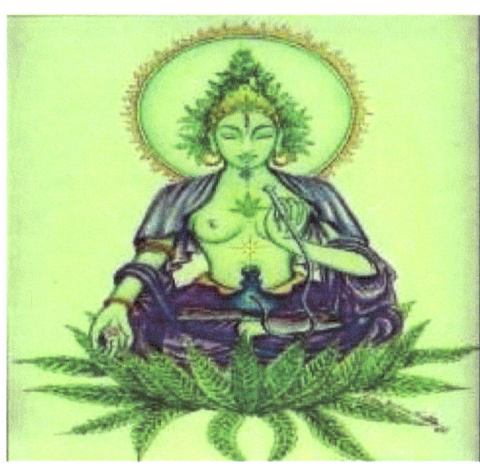

Hemp in Tibetan Medicine

"Buddhists consume Cannabis in order to obtain a mystical experience; the primary goal which is detachment from worldly things. Hemp has been an enduring component of the Tibetan pharmacopoeias since ancient times. Hemp seeds and the oil they yield (not to be confused with hash oil) are an important source of nutrition. In addition, rope and paper are manufactured from the fibers."

"Tibetans consider hemp to be a sacred plant, and they often cultivate it in proximity to monasteries and courtyards. In the Lamaistic tradition, it is said that Buddha nourished himself with just one hemp seed a day during the six ascetic years before his enlightenment. As a result, hemp seeds are an important food for fasting ascetics. Books in monasteries have been printed on hemp paper since the adoption of Buddhism."

In Tantric Buddhism, psychoactive hemp drinks continue to be used when meditating on the cosmic union of Buddha and his shakti as well as for the actual physical union between temple servants and priests. Here, the aphrodisiac cannabis is regarded as the "food of Kundalini", the female subtle creative energy that transforms sexual energy into spiritual experience. The drink is consumed 1 and 1/2 hours prior to meditation or the sexual yab/yum ritual so that the accumulation of its effects occurs at the beginning of the spiritual or physical activity.

In the Buddhist Tara Tantra, Cannabis is used as a rasayana, meaning an elixir of vitality. In the Tibetan Tara tantra, Cannabis is "essential to ecstasy".

Reference: Marijuana Medicine by Christian Ratsch pages 42 – 49

Cannabis in Chinese Medicine: The first recorded use of cannabis as a medicinal drug occurred in 2737 B.C. by Chinese emperor Shen Nung, father of Chinese medicine and acupuncture and author of Divine Husbandman's Materia Medica, the earliest extant Chinese pharmacopoeia. The emperor documented the drug's effectiveness in treating the pain of rheumatism and gout.

NOTE by Ricardo B Serrano: As a Chinese medicine and Qigong practitioner, I find that Cannabis is both an herbal medicine and an entheogenic substance used for healing and awakening our inner divinity via meditation/ Qigong.

References: Pot Brownie Recipe, page 18; How Cannabis works, page 19; Holistic Biochemistry of Cannabinoids, page 20; Endocannabinoid Deficiency, page 112; and Cannabis, acupuncture and Qigong, page 113

Cancer and Cannabis Medicines

In studies of cancer cells and some animal models, cannabinoids have been shown to inhibit tumor growth through a variety of mechanisms, though this antitumor activity has not yet been consistently demonstrated in human clinical trials. The effects include suppression of cancer cell signaling mechanisms, inhibition of both blood vessel growth to the tumor and cancer cell migration, and stimulation of programmed cell death in the cancer cell.

Cannabis medicines can stimulate appetite, encourage sleep, reduce anxiety and depression, elevate mood, treat nausea and vomiting, and reduce cancer pain.

A rule of thumb for Cannabis Dosage: Use the smallest possible dose required to meet the medicinal need, then set the shortest possible treatment course at that dosage in order to reduce the chance of a patient developing dose-tolerance issues. High doses can cause an imbalance of the endocannabinoid system, and the body therefore adjusts by reducing cannabinoid receptor density.

Effectiveness

- Nausea and vomiting
- Appetite stimulation - The endocannabinoid system regulates appetite.
- Pain - Cannabis medicines are quite effective for reducing, and even preventing, some forms of cancer pain.
- Sleep - Cannabis medicine can effectively encourage sleep in cancer patients.
- Mood elevation - The endocannabinoid system regulates mood.
- Anxiety and depression
- Antitumor activity

Methods of Ingestion

- **Oral**: Sublingual and swallowed forms are quite effective, but sublingual has a quicker onset and is more predictable. Swallowed medicines tend to provide longer-lasting effects and seem to have some advantages for nausea and vomiting, provided they are taken three hours before a chemo session.
- **Vaporization and smoking**: Vaporization is quite effective and titration of dose is easily achieved. In Israel, it is not uncommon to see patients vaporizing or even smoking cannabis during chemotherapy session.
- **Indicated chemotypes**: Typically broad-leafleted varieties high in myrcene, limonene, and linalool are recommended. CBD chemotypes are also useful for anxiety.
- **Popular varieties**: Nearly all varieties of cannabis will address the adverse effects stemming from cancer treatments. In particular, Cannatonic for its CBD content; and OG Kush, Grand Daddy Purple, Pincher Creek, and Bubba Kush for their THC and terpene content.

Reference: Cannabis Pharmacy Practical Guide to Medical Marijuana by Michael Backes, 2014, pages 191 – 194
References: Pot Brownie Recipe and Green Dragon Tincture, page 18; Endocannabinoid Deficiency, page 112; Cannabis, acupuncture and Qigong, page 113; How Cannabinoids Kill Cancer, page 132; Final Notes, page 134

NOTE by Ricardo B Serrano: As far as chemotherapy treatment is concerned, it is up to the choice of the patient to combine chemotherapy with cannabis or not since cannabis use alone is effective by itself therapeutically.

Popular Cannabis Varieties (Strains)

Grand Daddy Purple is described by the California dispensary as "The King of the Purps." This is the strain that many of the other purps were bred from. It is the ultimate calmative, sedative medicine and often used for pain relief. It is also indicated for treating insomnia, appetite stimulation, and spasticity.

The tested sample was analyzed at 18% THC. It had an acrid odor with a faint synthetic grape taste similar to grape soda. We surmised that it contained significant amounts of pinene, limonene, borneol and contained moderate levels of myrcene and terpenol. The feeling was very pleasant, relaxed and clearheaded, but none of us felt high.

OG Kush is described by the dispensary as:

"The first shock wave hits hard. It doesn't take long to realize that you're already feeling its effects from just one or two hits. A few puffs and the effects are long lasting and intense, but beware that the recovery period is prolonged. This bud is more of a late night adventure than a midday smoke break...It is a good strain for treating social anxiety, stress, depression and for appetite stimulation."

The sample we tested had 34% THC. It had a musky odor, almost like smelly feet and earthy. In addition it had floral tones, and cut lawn and sage odors. We surmised that it contained large amounts of myrcene, limonene, pinene, borneol and moderate amounts of linalool and pulgone. The high was friendly, mind opening and meditative. It took us to "new places."

Purple Kush is described by the dispensary as:

- "Its pain relieving effects are immediate. It's good for anxiety, depression, chronic pain, insomnia, stress and stomach disorders. The Kush high is a deep stone.
- "Its deep body stone delivers treatment for chronic pain, depression, insomnia, stress and stomach disorders.
- "The buds have a soft pine bouquet and a sweet, grapey taste on an earthy foundation. It has an indica taste."
- The high was "generic," it had no character. We felt it was sort of neutral which had 29% THC.

Marijuana Myths

- Marijuana impairs fertility and reproduction.
- Marijuana causes brain damage.
- Marijuana use leads to chromosome and cell damage.
- Marijuana damages the immune system.
- Marijuana offers a "gateway" to hard drug abuse.
- Marijuana use causes violence.
  Real Concerns include: (1) Long-term health effects of marijuana use - primarily damage from smoking and risk of accidental injury. (2) Mental impairment while under the influence.
  Reference: Marijuana Medical Handbook by Dale Gieringer, PhD, 2008, pages 116, 221 - 223

Before Using Cannabis

You must speak with your physician or healthcare professional before using medical cannabis, as the use of cannabis may not be safe for you, or special precautions may be advised if you suffer from:

- Schizophrenia, bipolar disorder, or severe depression
- Heart disease, high blood pressure, angina, or irregular heartbeat
- Chronic obstructive pulmonary disease
- An immune disorder

Younger patients should exercise significant caution before using THC-dominant cannabis medicines and consider using cannabis medicines with higher CBD to THC ratios.

Mild Adverse Effects of Medical Cannabis

- Rapid heartbeat, referred to as tachycardia. Rapid heartbeat typically subsides within 15 to 20 minutes. Slow, steady breathing for a few minutes can help while the racing heartbeat gradually begins to subside.
- Dry mouth, informally called "cottonmouth." Dry mouth can be addressed with water or, even better, lemonade. Lemonade with added lemon peel is a popular local remedy in North Africa to reduce the mild side effects of cannabis use.
- Dizziness or lightheadedness can seem less pronounced when the eyes are kept clean and focused on something, such as watching television.
- Red, irritated eyes can be treated using mild eyedrops, such as VISINE, which quickly relieve any itchy or burning eyes.
- Coughing caused by inhaled cannabis smoke or vapor is rarely dangerous and usually subsides quickly. It is most easily avoided by simply reducing the amount inhaled. A glass of water can also help. Care must be taken when inhaling concentrated forms of cannabis, such as cannabis resin (hashish) or oil (hash oil, butter, wax, or dabs), since too much can result in a brutal coughing fit that can damage the lungs. If airway irritation becomes an issue with inhaled cannabis, then oral or sublingual cannabis administration methods should be explored.

None of the listed side effects is immediate cause for alarm, but calming someone who is experiencing any one of them for the first time can be quite a challenge.

The use of cannabis during pregnancy and breast-feeding cannot be recommended.

Additionally, cannabis medicines (smoked, oral, sublingual, or vaporized) increase the effects of alcohol, benzodiazepines (Ativan, Halcion, Librium, Restoril, Valium, Xanax, etc.) and opiates (codeine, fentanyl, morphine, etc.).

References: Cannabis Pharmacy by Michael Backes, 2014, pages 35 – 37, and Stoned by D. Casarett, MD

References: Pot Brownie Recipe and Green Dragon Tincture, page 18; Endocannabinoid Deficiency, page 112; Cannabis, and Qigong, page 113; How Cannabinoids Kill Cancer, page 132; Final Notes, page 134

NOTE: Cachexia and cancer, elaborated in the following articles, can be treated by the use of medical cannabis (cannabis hemp) instead of hydrazine sulfate. Medical cannabis reduces pain and helps cancer patients sleep and rest. It reduces nausea and vomiting caused by chemotherapy. It stimulates their appetites to help them eat and combat excessive weight loss (wasting syndrome) - cachexia. It also usually raises the patients' spirits, mood and will to live, improving their overall chances of recovery.

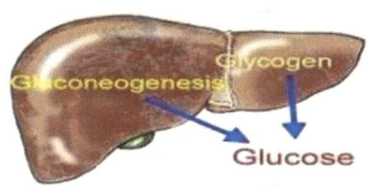

What causes cachexia in cancer?

Cancer has two principal devastating effects on the body. One is the invasion of the tumor into the vital organs, with the destruction of the organ's functions - the most common cause of death in the public's mind. In reality, however, this accounts for only about 23 percent of the country's half-million annual cancer deaths.

The other devastating effect of cancer is cachexia, the terrible wasting away of the body, with its attendant weight loss and debilitation. In cancer, as in AIDS, patients succumb to the accompanying illnesses, which they would otherwise survive if not for the wasting syndrome.

"In a sense, nobody ever dies of cancer," notes Dr. Harold Dvorak, chief of pathology at Beth Israel Hospital in Boston. "They die of something else - pneumonia, failure of one or other organs. Cachexia accelerates that process of infection and the building-up of metabolic poisons. It causes death a lot faster than the tumor would, were it not for the cachexia.

Halting the wasting syndrome instead of directly attacking the cancer cells with poison was Dr. Gold's plan of attack. As he explains. "Each of these processes [the tumor invasion of vital organs and cachexia] has its own metabolic machinery, each is amenable to its own therapy, and each is to some degree functionally interdependent of the other. In the interest of treating the totality of malignant disease, each of these processes warrants intervention. Such an approach, dealing with both major underpinnings of the cancerous process - mitogenic and metabolic - affords the greatest promise of eliciting long-term, symptom-free survival and the potential for disease eradication."

But what causes cachexia? Cancer cells gobble up sugar ten to fifteen times more than normal cells do. The sugar consumed by the cancer cells is generated mainly from the liver, which converts lactic acid into glucose. (Normal cells are far more efficient users of glucose, which they derive from the food we eat, not from lactic acid.) When cancer cells use sugar (glucose) as fuel, they only partially metabolize it. Lactic acid - the waste product of this incomplete combustion - spills into the blood and is taken up by the liver. The liver then recycles the lactic acid (and other breakdown products) back into glucose, and the sugar is consumed in ever-increasing amounts by voracious cancer cells. The result is a vicious cycle, what Dr. Gold calls a "sick relationship" between the liver and cancer. The patient's healthy cells starve while the cancer cells grow vigorously. Some healthy cells even dissolve to feed the growing tumor.

To break this sick relationship, Gold reasoned, all he needed was to find a safe, nontoxic drug that inhibits gluconeogenesis (the liver's recycling of lactic acid into glucose). In 1968, he outlined his theory in an article published in Oncology. "The silence was deafening," he recalls.

A year later, by a remarkable coincidence, Gold heard biochemist Paul Ray deliver a paper explaining that hydrazine sulfate could shut down the enzyme necessary for the production of glucose from lactic acid. Gold had chanced upon an eminently logical way of starving cancer. He immediately tested hydrazine sulfate on mice and found that in accord with his theory, the drug inhibited both gluconeogenesis and tumor growth...

Approximately half of the patients to whom the drug is properly administered in the early stages of the disease show an almost immediate weight gain and reversal of symptoms; in some instances, the tumor eventually disappears. The most common types of cancer most frequently reported to benefit from hydrazine sulfate therapy are recto-colon cancer, ovarian cancer, prostatic cancer, lung (bronchogenic) cancer, Hodgkin's disease and other lymphomas, thyroid cancer, melanoma, and breast cancer. Some less common types of cancer also benefit...

The wasting syndrome seen in cancer patients is also a prime risk factor for AIDS patients with Kaposi's sarcoma. There is evidence that hydrazine sulfate's capacity to stop cachexia may save many AIDS patients. Currently, Dr. Chlebowski is planning a study to test hydrazine sulfate as an anticachexia agent in patients who are infected with HIV and have lost weight...

Source: Options: the Alternative Cancer Therapy Book by Richard Walters, 1993. pages 49-53

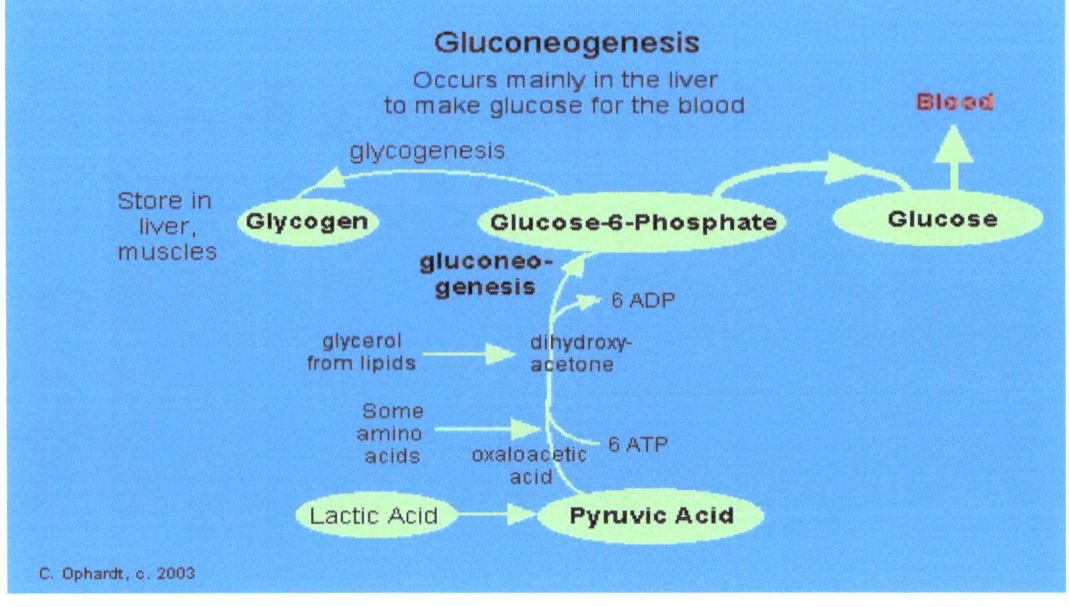

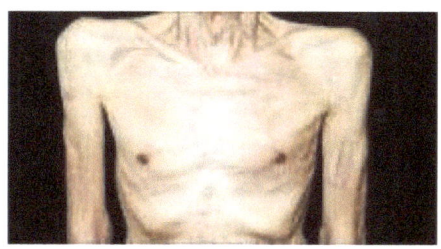

Cachexia in Cancer/ AIDS

Hydrazine Sulfate: Unorthodox Chemotherapy

Hydrazine sulfate therapy is a new type of chemotherapy (Gold, 1975).

Dr. Joseph Gold, MD, of Syracuse, New York, reasoned that cachexia is but the end result of an insidious process - unrecognizable at first, but slowly taking its toll of the body's reserves until a "point of no return" is reached. Cachexia begins with the very first cancer tissue. What we need is a way to stop the vicious cycle and thereby put a halt to the leading cause of death in cancer: cachexia (Gold, 1968).

Soviet scientists seemed to grasp the philosophical basis of Gold's new approach better than his own countrymen. They wrote:

Almost all research in the field of experimental and clinical chemotherapy of malignant neoplasia [cancer] up to the present time, one way or another, reflects the principles of a direct ... attack on growth and multiplication of cancer cells. However, there may well be other means of medicinal influence on the progress of neoplastic growth. One of these includes Gold's hypothesis (Seits et al., 1975).

The Soviet team confirm the following claims for hydrazine therapy:

Hydrazine stops the growth of animal cancers: Soviet scientists found that hydrazine definitely retards the growth of cancer in experimental animals. In Walker carcinosarcoma in rats, for instance, they were able to demonstrate a 97.4 percent inhibition of tumor growth with a high dose of hydrazine given orally. Other types of experimental cancer also showed moderate response to the drug. (ibid.)

Hydrazine works by stopping gluconeogenesis: This, at least, was the most likely explanation of the drug's action. Microscopic examination of tumor remnants in cured rats showed "well-preserved tumor tissues." This means that hydrazine destroys tumors without directly poisoning cancer cells by some "indirect mechanism of inhibition of tumor growth." (ibid.)

Hydrazine is relatively nontoxic: In animals, there was no damage to the liver of the treated animals, and little weight loss, especially at lower dosage levels. Most important, in humans there was no damage to the blood-making cells, although in a minority of patients the Soviet doctors saw the same minor side effects as Gold noted, such as limb weakness and nausea. (ibid.)

Hydrazine controls cancerous growths in humans: This is of course the bottom line of any cancer therapy. Forty-eight patients were given hydrazine as a last resort "in all cases after exhausting possibilities of surgical, X-ray treatment or other types of chemotherapy." In other words, these were patients on whom nothing else would work - patients with debilitated bodies, doomed to die within a few months. (ibid.)

The Soviet scientists carefully followed Gold's suggestions for dosages. They noted that the usual criteria for evaluation of the effectiveness of a drug - especially tumor shrinkage - may not be applicable in this case "in view of the unusual action of hydrazine sulfate." Nevertheless, in these forty-eight very sick, terminal patients the Russians achieved the following results:

Objective anticancer effects in over one-third of the patients tested: This included "objective regressions of tumor mass" in 20 percent of the cases and an additional 15 percent whose cases were stabilized: i.e., whose cancers stopped progressing.

Subjective anticancer effects in 58 percent of the patients: This included complete disappearance or marked reduction of bone pain, increase in appetite, and an unexpected desire to get out of their beds and walk around. In short, there was a "sharp improvement of general well-being" in over half the terminal patients. (ibid.)

The Soviet scientists found that hydrazine was not simply a painkiller in the ordinary sense, but induced a sense of euphoria in many patients. Suddenly people who were in the doldrums, waiting to die, became active, cheerful, optimistic, wanting to live. The Soviet doctors noted hydrazine sulfate's "peculiar influence on the psyche," particularly a "sharp improvement of mood in a significant portion of the patients ... to the point of euphoria" (Danova et al. 1977). This was so even in cases where no objective regression of the cancer could be seen.

In 1981 the Russian team, headed by Gershanovich, finally found an American outlet for their complete pro-hydrazine results. They reported in a new journal, Nutrition and Cancer, that the drug had a marked and dramatic effect on the symptoms and disease progression of cancer patients (Gershanovich, 1981).

"A clear-cut statement for hydrazine sulfate as an anticachexia agent can be made," the Russians concluded (ibid.).

In the wake of such studies, in Novembber 1979 the American Cancer Society removed hydrazine from its unproven methods list. Dr. G. Congdon Wood of the ACS was quoted as saying that hydrazine sulfate "shows great promise as a tool doctors can use to ease symptoms of cancer (Miami Herald, November 23, 1981)

Behind the scenes, however, continued a fierce struggle on how to deal with the drug. In fact, the cancer world split, not just over hydrazine sulfate, but over the value of anti-cachexia agents in general. Some scientists, like Gold, put their focus on restoring the health of the patient's metabolism. His drug was a way of helping the body fight its cancer and, in so doing, slow down tumor growth. Others were fixated on dramatic cures, the elusive kind of breakthroughs symbolized at that moment by much-heralded interferon. It was a profound philosophical divide.

"I believe that cachexia is a major problem in dealing with oncology today," said Dr. Gio Gori. Gori had left NCI because of its neglect of nutritional issues. He became the founding editor of Nutrition and Cancer (Moss, 1983).

Nearly twenty years after it was proposed, despite numerous positive tests including three positive double-blind studies - hydrazine is still unaccepted by the mainstream.

"NCI is up to its usual tricks," Gold reflects. "What it couldn't do in the scientific arena, it is trying to accomplish through politics" (Gold, 1988).

At this writing, the Syracuse Cancer Research Institute is once again facing financial hardships. There is not enough research funding to do the necessary work. Why? Gold played by the rules. He did not profiteer from patients. He did not organize supporters to march on Washington, turn his back on the scientific method, or run away to exotic tropical islands. He won his twenty year battle for hydrazine but now stands in danger of losing the war. His very success has been turned against him. By an adroit use of "repressive tolerance" the cancer establishment has simultaneously tried to neutralize hydrazine sulfate's threat while grabbing credit for its open-minded acceptance of new ideas.

*Seits, I. F., et al. "Experimental and Critical Data of Antitumor Action of Hydrazine Sulfate." Problems of Oncology (Leningrad) 21:45-52, 1975.

*Gershanovich, M. L.; Danova, L. A.: Ivin, B. A.; and Filov, V. A. "Results of Clinical Study of Antitumor Action of Hydrazine Sulfate." Nutrition and Cancer 3:7-12, 1981.

Source: The Cancer Industry: The Classic Expose on the Cancer Establishment by Ralph W. Moss, 1989. pages 196-198, 204-205.

Hydrazine sulfate is an anti-cachexia drug which acts to reverse the metabolic processes of debilitation and weight loss in cancer and secondarily acts to stabilize and regress tumors. Hydrazine sulfate is a monoamine oxidase (MAO) inhibitor and is incompatible with tranquilizers, barbiturates, alcohol and other central nervous system depressants. Foods high in tyramine, such as aged cheeses and fermented products, are also incompatible with MAO inhibitors. The use of tranquilizers, barbiturates and/or alcoholic beverages with hydrazine sulfate destroys the efficacy of this drug and increases patient morbidity.

HYDRAZINE SULFATE's original proponent, Dr. Joseph Gold of the Syracuse Cancer Research Institute of New York has been fighting years for acceptance of this virtually side effect free, non- toxic therapy despite the reluctance of more rigid, conventionally entrenched, orthodox practitioners who now may be taking another look at the results in both America and abroad.

Brand Name for Hydrazine Sulfate: Sehydrin by Pharmsynthez

The use of tranquilizers, barbiturates and/or alcoholic beverages with hydrazine sulfate destroys the efficacy of this drug and increases patient morbidity.

Hydrazine Sulfate is given to cancer patients on a specific formula.

One (1) capsule/tablet per day, 1/2 (half) hours before a meal, for three (3) days. (total 3 capsules/tablets)

On the 4th day increase dosage to two (2) capsules/tablets per day, for four (4) days (Total 8 capsules/tablets for the four day period).am/pm

On the 8th day increase dosage by one (1) capsule/tablet per day. (total capsules/tablets at this point is 3 per day).am/noon/pm

ALWAYS TAKE THE CAPSULES ON EMPTY STOMACH, just before your meal.

Upon completion of the first 100 units (capsules/tablets), wait seven (7) days before beginning the next bottle. With the second or following bottles of capsules/tablets, the maintenance dosage is two (2) tablets per day. am/pm

MAXIMUM RECOMMENDED DOSAGE is 3 capsules/tablets in any 24 hour period, but may be adjusted on advice by your health care professional.

When taking Hydrazine Sulfate the use of any alcohol and/or barbiturates is PROHITED. This includes prescription pain medication. Consult your personal health care professional to qualify any other medication you may be taking.

ALWAYS CONSULT YOUR PERSONAL PHYSICIAN/HEALTH CARE PROFESSIONAL BEFORE TAKING ANY MEDICATION.

Minor Side Effects: (Contraindications) It is possible, under long term usage of high dosages, a small percentage of patients may experience some temporary mild extremity numbness, nausea and/or occasional drowsiness. The symptoms usually disappear within days.

Recommended Dosage/Potency is determined by bodyweight:

* Patient under 55KG (125 lb) -- 30 mg

* Patient over 55KG (125+lb) - 60 mg

In Canada: 604-856-0171 Life Energy Distributor

http://store.lifepharma.com

In summary, the following things should not be taken with Hydrazine Sulphate:

1. ethanol
2. alcoholic beverages
3. barbiturates and tranquilizers (e.g. Thorazine, Compazine, Xanax, Valium, Dalmane, Ativan, Restoril, Halcion, Nembutal and Seconal, to name but a few)
4. sedatives in doses greater than 100 mg per day, especially benzodiazepines and phenothiazines
5. antihistamines
6. antiemetics
7. other agents that depress the central nervous system, such as morphine
8. foods with tyramine
9. Vitamin B6
10. Vitamin C in daily doses above 250 mg (from all sources)

Tyramine-Rich Foods

Please review the dietary restrictions that should be observed when a patient is receiving monoamine oxidase inhibitor (MAOI) therapy?

R. Tyramine, is an amino acid which is found in various foods, and is an indirect sympathomimetic that can cause a hypertensive reaction in patients receiving MAOI therapy. Monoamine oxidase is found in the gastrointestinal tract and inactivates tyramine; when drugs prevent the catabolism of exogenous tyramine, this amino acid is absorbed and displaces norepinephrine from sympathetic nerve ending and epinephrine from the adrenal glands. If a sufficient amount of pressor amines are released, a patient may experience a severe occipital or temporal headache, diaphoresis, mydriasis, nuchal rigidity, palpitations, and the elevation of both diastolic and systolic blood pressure may ensue (Anon, 1989; Da Prada et al, 1988; Brown & Bryant, 1988). On rare occasions, cardiac arrhythmias, cardiac failure, and intracerebral hemorrhage have developed in patients receiving MAOI therapy that did not observe dietary restrictions (Brown & Bryant, 1988). Therefore, dietary restrictions are required for patients receiving MAOIs. Extensive dietary restrictions previously published were collected over a decade ago and due to changes in food processing and more reliable analytical methods, new recommendations have been published (Anon, 1989; McCabe, 1986). The tyramine content of foods varies greatly due to the differences in processing, fermentation, ripening, degradation, or incidental contamination. Many foods contain small amounts of tyramine and the formation of large quantities of tyramine have been reported if products were aged, fermented, or left to spoil. Because the sequela from tyramine and MAOIs is dose-related, reactions can be minimized without total abstinence from tyramine-containing foods. Approximately 10 to 25 mg of tyramine is required for a severe reaction compared to 6 to 10 mg for a mild reaction. Foods that normally contain low amounts of tyramine may become a risk if unusually large quantities are consumed or if spoilage has occurred (McCabe, 1986). Three lists were compiled (foods to avoid, foods that may used in small quantities, and foods with insufficient evidence to restrict) to minimized the strict dietary restrictions that were previously used and improve compliance and safety of MAOI therapy. The foods to avoid list consists of foods with sufficient tyramine (in small or usual serving sizes) that would create a dangerous elevation in blood pressure and therefore should be avoided (McCabe, 1986)

Foods to Avoid

ALCOHOLIC BEVERAGES - avoid Chianti wine and vermouth. Consumption of red, white, and port WINE in quantities less than 120 mL present little risk (Anon, 1989; Da Prada et al, 1988; McCabe, 1986). BEER and ALE should also be avoided (McCabe, 1986), however other investigators feel major domestic (US) brands of beer is safe in small quantities (1/2 cup or less than 120 mL) (Anon, 1989; Da Prada, 1988), but imported beer should not be consumed unless a specific brand is known to be safe. WHISKEY and LIQUEURS such as Drambuie(R) and Chartreuse(R) have caused reactions. NONALCOHOLIC BEVERAGES (alcohol- free beer and wines) may contain tyramine and should be avoided (Anon, 1989; Stockley, 1993).

BANANA PEELS - a single case report implicates a BANANA as the causative agent, which involved the consumption of whole stewed green banana, including the peel. Ripe banana pulp contains 7 mcg/gram of tyramine compared to a peel which contains 65 mcg/gram and 700 mcg of tyramine and dopamine, respectively (McCabe, 1986).

BEAN CURD - fermented bean curd, fermented soya bean, soya bean pastes contain a significant amount of tyramine (Anon, 1989).

BROAD (FAVA) BEAN PODS - these beans contain dopa, not tyramine, which is metabolized to dopamine and may cause a pressor reaction and therefore should not be eaten particularly if overripe (McCabe, 1986; Anon, 1989; Brown & Bryant, 1988).

CHEESE - tyramine content cannot be predicted based on appearance, flavor, or variety and therefore should be avoided. CREAM CHEESE and COTTAGE CHEESE have no detectable level of tyramine (McCabe, 1986; Anon, 1989, Brown & Bryant, 1988).

FISH - fresh fish (Anon, 1989; McCabe, 1986) and vacuum- packed pickled fish or CAVIAR contain only small amounts of tyramine and are safe if consumed promptly or refrigerated for short periods; longer storage may be dangerous (Anon, 1989). Smoked, fermented, pickled (Herring) and otherwise aged fish, meat, or any spoiled food may contain high levels of tyramine and should be avoided (Anon, 1989; Brown & Bryant, 1988).

GINSENG - some preparations have resulted in a headache, tremulousness, and manic-like symptoms (Anon, 1989).

PROTEIN EXTRACTS - three brands of meat extract contained 95, 206, and 304 mcg/gram of tyramine and therefore meat extracts should be avoided (McCabe, 1986). Avoid liquid and powdered PROTEIN DIETARY SUPPLEMENTS (Anon, 1989).

MEAT, nonfresh or liver - no detectable levels identified in fresh chicken livers; high tyramine content found in spoiled or unfresh livers (McCabe, 1986). Fresh meat is safe, caution suggested in restaurants (Anon, 1989; Da Prada et al, 1988).

SAUSAGE, BOLOGNA, PEPPERONI and SALAMI contain large amounts of tyramine (Anon, 1989; Da Prada et al, 1988; McCabe, 1986). No detectable tyramine levels were identified in country CURED HAM (McCabe, 1986).

SAUERKRAUT - tyramine content has varied from 20 to 95 mcg/gram and should be avoided (McCabe, 1986).

SHRIMP PASTE - contain a large amount of tyramine (Anon, 1989).

SOUPS - should be avoided as protein extracts may be present; miso soup is prepared from fermented bean curd and contain tyramine in large amounts and should not be consumed (Anon, 1989).

YEAST, Brewer's or extracts - yeast extracts (Marmite) which are spread on bread or mixed with water, Brewer's yeast, or yeast vitamin supplements should not be consumed. Yeast used in baking is safe (Anon, 1989; Da Prada et al, 1988; McCabe, 1986).

The foods to use with caution list categorizes foods that have been reported to cause a hypertensive crisis if foods were consumed in large quantities, stored for prolong periods, or if contamination occurred. Small servings (1/2 cup, or less than 120 mL) of the following foods are not expected to pose a risk for patients on MAOI therapy (McCabe, 1986).

FOODS TO USE WITH CAUTION

(1/2 cup or less than 120 mL)

Alcoholic beverages - see under foods to avoid.

AVOCADOS - contain tyramine, particularly overripe (Anon, 1989) but may be used in small amounts if not overripened (McCabe, 1986).

CAFFEINE - contains a weak pressor agent, large amounts may cause a reaction (Anon, 1989).

CHOCOLATE - is safe to ingest for most patients, unless consumed in large amounts (Anon, 1989; McCabe, 1986).

DAIRY PRODUCTS - CREAM, SOUR CREAM, cottage cheese, cream cheese, YOGURT, or MILK should pose little risk unless prolonged storage or lack of sanitation standards exists (Anon, 1989; McCabe, 1986). Products should not be used if close to the expiration date (McCabe, 1986).

NUTS - large quantities of PEANUTS were implicated in a hypertensive reaction and headache. COCONUTS and BRAZIL NUTS have also been implicated, however no analysis of the tyramine content was performed (McCabe, 1986).

RASPBERRIES - contain tyramine and small amounts are expected to be safe (McCabe, 1986).

SOY SAUCE - has been reported to contain large amounts of tyramine and reactions have been reported with teriyaki (Anon, 1989), however analysis of soy sauce reveals a tyramine level of 1.76 mcg/mL and fermented meat may have contributed to the previously reported reactions (McCabe, 1986).

SPINACH, New Zealand prickly or hot weather - large amounts have resulted in a reaction (Anon, 1989; McCabe, 1986).

More than 200 foods contain tyramine in small quantities and have been implicated in reactions with MAOI therapy, however the majority of the previous reactions were due to the consumption of spoiled food. Evidence does not support the restriction of the following foods listed if the food is fresh (McCabe, 1986).

FOODS WITH INSUFFICIENT EVIDENCE FOR RESTRICTION (McCabe, 1986)

anchovies - cream cheese - raisins

   beetroot - cucumbers - salad dressings

   chips with vinegar - egg, boiled - snails

   Coca Cola(R) - figs, canned - tomato juice

   cockles - fish, canned - wild game

   coffee - junket - worcestershire sauce

   corn, sweet - mushrooms - yeast-leavened bread

   cottage cheese - pineapple, fresh

Any protein FOOD, improperly stored or handled, can form pressor amines through protein breakdown. Chicken and beef liver, liver pate, and game generally contain high amine levels due to frequent mishandling. Game is often allowed to partially decompose as part of its preparation. Ayd (1986) reported that the freshness of the food is a key issue with MAOIs and that as long as foods are purchased from reputable shops and stored properly, the danger of a hypertensive crisis is minimal. Some foods should be avoided, the most dangerous being aged cheeses and yeast products used as food supplements (Gilman et al, 1985).

With appropriate dietary restrictions, the incidence of hypertensive crises has decreased to approximately 4% (Zisook, 1985). Treatment of a hypertensive reactions includes the=7F administration of phentolamine (Anon, 1989) 2.5 to 5 milligrams intravenously (slow) titrated against blood pressure (Zisook,=7F 1985; Lippman & Nash, 1990). One report has suggested that the use of sublingual nifedipine 10 milligrams was effective in treating 2 hypertensive reactions following the ingestion of a tyramine-containing food in a patient receiving MAOI therapy (Clary & Schweizerr, 1987). Chlorpromazine also has alpha-blocking properties and has been recommended as an agent for discretionary use (patient-initiated treatment) in the setting of dietary indiscretion (Lippman & Nash, 1990).

CONCLUSION:

Dietary restrictions are required for individuals receiving monoamine oxidase inhibitor therapy to prevent a hypertensive crisis and other side effects. The foods listed in the dietary restrictions have been categorized into those foods that must be avoided, foods that may be ingested in small quantities, and those foods that were previous implicated in reactions but upon analyses of fresh samples only a small tyramine content was identified and should be safe to consume if freshness is considered.

REFERENCES:

1. Anon: Foods interacting with MAOI inhibitors. Med Lett Drug Ther 1989; 31:11-12.
2. Ayd FJ: Diet and monoamine oxidase inhibitors (MAOIs): an update. Int Drug Ther Newslett 1986; 21:19-20.
3. Brown CS & Bryant SG: Monoamine oxidase inhibitors: safety and efficacy issues. Drug Intell Clin Pharm 1988; 22:232-235.
4. Clary C & Schweizer E: Treatment of MAOI hypertensive crisis with sublingual nifedipine. J Clin Psychiatry 1987; 48:249-250.
5. Da Prada M, Zurcher G, Wuthrich I et al: On tyramine, food, beverages and the reversible MAO inhibitor moclobemide. J Neural Transm 1988; 26(Suppl):31-56.
6. Gilman AG, Goodman LS & Rall TW et al (Ed): Goodman and Gilman's The Pharmacological Basis of Therapeutics, 7th ed., Macmillan Publishing, New York, NY, 1985.
7. Lippman SB & Nash K: Monoamine oxidase inhibitor update. Potential adverse food and drug interactions. Drug Safety 1990; 5:195-204.
8. McCabe BJ: Dietary tyramine and other pressor amines in MAOI regimens: a review. J Am Diet Assoc 1986; 86:1059-1064.
9. Stockley I: Alcohol-free beer not safe for MAOI patients. Pharm J 1993; 250:174.
10. Zisook S: A clinical overview of monoamine oxidase inhibitors. Psychosomatics 1985; 26:240-251.

AUTHOR INFORMATION:

Theodore G Tong, Pharm D/C Hansen

Assistant Clinical Professor of Pharmacy

University of California

San Franscisco, California 94143

10/79 Revised by DRUGDEX(R) Editorial Staff, Denver, Colorado 80204: 09/82; 09/83; 07/85; 07/86; 09/89; 04/93; 01/94 (DC2763)

Stephen R. Saklad, Pharm.D. - saklad@uthscsa.edu

Psychiatric Pharmacy Program

The Univ Texas College of Pharmacy

(210) 567-8355 (Voice), (210) 567-8328 (FAX)

Testimonials on Medical Cannabis

"Cannabis with Qigong is the main herb that took care of my left eye pain together with my other symptoms such as sciatic pain, fatigue, high blood pressure and depression." – Ricardo B Serrano

"If I hadn't had the cannabis to get through the nauseousness, I would have lost weight and, I don't know, who knows what would have happened."

"Cannabis gives me a lift. It doesn't lay me back or anything. I want to do things, and it gave me energy that I didn't have at that time. I could eat. That was the important thing." - Brenda L. of Ohio: Breast Cancer

But she still talks to people about cannabis; those diagnosed with cancer. If they can't eat or can't sleep – "I know it will help them." - Catherine Adaberry of Missouri: Breast Cancer

Testimonials on Hydrazine Sulfate

"The most remarkable anticancer agent I have come across in my 45 years experience in cancer."— Dean Burk, M.D. at the time head of cell chemistry research at the NCI in the 1970's.

"Hydrazine sulfate, a drug that costs about a dollar a day, reverses the devastating weight loss called cachexia that kills most cancer patients. This simple chemical, developed in 1969 by Dr. Joseph Gold, director or the Syracuse Cancer Institute, works in half of all the patients who take it. Yet more than two million cancer patients starve to death yearly because the National Cancer Institute (NCI) continues its 20-year suppression of this life-saving drug. Meanwhile, doctors at the Petrov Institute of Oncology in St. Petersburg treating 1,000 patients with hydazine sulfate report long-term survival even in those with lymphatic cancer, the type that killed Jacqueline Onassis."— Dr. Julian Whitaker, M.D.

"True to an apparent mission of preventing effective cancer cures from being discovered, NCI worked skilfully to discredit hydrazine sulfate and to keep any knowledge from the general public."—John Diamond.

"NCI's actions with respect to hydrazine sulfate, characterized by intimidation, coercion, steadfast opposition, and possibly clinical trial-rigging, are truly one of the most shameful, scandalous medical undertakings in this country's history, depriving vast numbers of people of their health, happiness, and lives." Dr Gold

Joanne Daniloff D.VM.D., and professor at Louisiana State University in Baton Rouge, explained in a letter to Jeff Camen in 1994 how hydrazine sulfate had saved her life. At the time, she had survived 7 years after receiving surgery and hydrazine sulfate for her glioblastoma multiforme (grade 4) brain cancer, one of the fastest growing and most untreatable kinds (about 1% survival with orthodox therapies). "You understand, then, that I am appalled by the (NCI's) design of studies that result in claims that hydrazine sulfate has little or no effect on cancer treatment. I find it difficult to understand how any study with such obvious flaws can claim any result or be published in any reputable journal." (ref John Diamond)

Dr. Joseph Gold speaks....

If you have cancer, even advanced, studies show this drug may help save your life....

A year ago, on February 21, 2008, I placed a blog on MedTruth, "A Dog Has a Better Chance of Recovering from Cancer Than You Do," in which I attempted to show, in dramatic fashion, that the public is being "hoodwinked" from using hydrazine sulfate for human cancer, principally by the U.S. National Cancer Institute--part of the federal government--whereas the veterinary industry is largely immune from this constraint, using hydrazine sulfate on animals sick with cancer, many of whom, as a result of this treatment, are being reported to have staged significant or complete recovery. I went on in this blog to show that it was our National Cancer Institute (NCI) which was knowingly spreading misinformation on this drug to the public and to the medical profession, in an attempt to keep it from becoming adopted for routine use in human malignancy.

The reason for the present blog is to emphasize the great possibilities for improvement and curative effect by this drug for individuals with cancers of almost all types--and at all stages--whether hydrazine sulfate is used by itself, with chemotherapy or radiation therapy, or with other modalities of cancer treatment, and eliminate, to the extent possible, the "contest" imposed on this drug by the NCI.

Controlled clinical trials, done in conformity with the Helsinki Declaration, show that of every million late-stage, unresponsive cancer patients treated with hydrazine sulfate, more than half a million would receive measurable symptomatic improvement, 400,000 would demonstrate a halt or regression in tumor growth, and some would go on to long term (>10 years) "complete response," i.e., survival.

These are truly late-stage patients--i.e., those who have become refractory to their treatments or were never responsive to them in the first place. (It would be expected that in "earlier" patients the foregoing very favorable results would be even improved.)

These clinical results emanate from 17 years of Phase II multicentric clinical trials headquartered at the Petrov Research Institute of Oncology in St. Petersburg (with participation of the Herzen Institute of Oncology, Moscow; Oncological Institute of Lithuania, Vilnius; Institute of Oncology of the Ukranian Academy of Sciences, Kiev; and Rostov Institute of Oncology and Radiology, Rostov-an Danou)-- and 10 years of randomized, double-blind Phase III clinical trials at Harbor-UCLA Medical Center in California, performed by scientists considered among the most outstanding and experienced clinical cancer investigators in the world and published chiefly in leading U.S. peer-reviewed cancer and scientific journals.

The Helsinki Declaration--an outgrowth of the Nuremberg Trials (Doctors Trial) following World War II which uncovered the hideous human medical "experiments" inflicted on helpless human beings by the Nazis--is a multinational ratification of principles governing human biomedical research studies, to which the U.S. is a major signatory, put in place to guarantee that no harmful procedures be used in patients undergoing experimental medical treatment. This document lies at the very heart of all clinical studies and informed consent--and as such represents the international "law of the land" and requires all human biomedical research to conform to its stated principles.

The only controlled clinical trials to find this drug non-effective were those sponsored by the U.S. National Cancer Institute--which were in violation of the Helsinki Declaration by their use of incompatible agents in the presence of a test drug. The paramount principle--Principle 1--of the Helsinki Declaration states: "Biomedical research involving human subjects must conform to generally accepted scientific principles...and be based on a thorough knowledge of the scientific literature." Most important of generally accepted scientific principles in the conduct of human biomedical research is that no incompatible agents (medications) be used in a drug trial, since such use can result in the grave illness-- or death--of a patient, as well as cause a negative drug study. Use of incompatible agents in a drug study is virtually unknown in human biomedical testing.

In the blog, "A Dog Has a Better Chance...." it was shown that the NCI-sponsored studies, out of conformity with the Helsinki Declaration by violation of the "generally accepted standards" rule (Principle 1), were also under the leadership of inexperienced or ethically compromised investigators, were not "juried" in the usual manner (it was not clear whether they were subject to outside, independent peer-review prior to publication), were "interconnected"--i.e., not independent of one another (thus no independent conformation was possible), and were subject to an accompanying NCI editorial containing blatant, unscientific language, referring to hydrazine sulfate as a "vampire," thus impairing their "legitimacy" as impartial, objective scientific investigations.

In contrast, the Petrov and Harbor-UCLA studies were in full compliance with the Helsinki Declaration, were carried out by experienced, world-class investigators not involved in any irregularities or conflicts of interest, were subject to outside, independent peer-review before winning publication, were not "interconnected" and thus constituted independent confirmation of one another (reinforcing the validity of their individual data). These studies were carried out in strict accordance with internationally established and recognized principles and contained no additions or modifications which might act to dilute or question their scientific, impartial, objective integrity.

It is important to note that while the NCI is the largest cancer agency in the world and its scientific opinions considered most authoritative and regarded by the medical profession in the highest repute, once a study is incompetently performed--in this case in violation of "generally accepted scientific principles," in violation of an international Agreement of principles governing allowable human biomedical research procedures, to which the United States is a signatory--it doesn't matter what the "credentials" of the sponsoring organization are or in what esteem it is held, its studies are invalid. Period. Science declares they are null and void and must be excluded from any treatment options.

There are only two sets of valid, controlled clinical trials--those which are in full compliance with the Helsinki Declaration--on hydrazine sulfate: the Russian (Petrov) and the Harbor-UCLA data. Both sets of studies show the same results: In late-stage patients who are or have become refractory to all treatments, hydrazine sulfate produces an approximate 50 percent response rate. 50 percent of these "factually terminal" patients respond with "moderate-to-marked" symptomatic improvements (decrease in weakness, pain and other cancer-specific symptoms, return of appetite, well-being), tumor stabilization (no tumor progression), tumor regression, or a combination of these effects. These benefits will persist from months to years, and in some cases will endure long term (>10 years), accompanied by complete response (total remission of disease).

These results are not a bad "scorecard" for those who have only "30 to 60" days to live, who are in the throes of weakness, pain and organ failure. The point is, there are no valid, controlled clinical data to disagree with these results.

Then why wouldn't--shouldn't--all patients with cancer want an immediate try on hydrazine sulfate? The results suggest that all unresponsive patients--or those growing weaker on their present therapy--who have no further treatment options available, should. Even earlier patients whose disease is stable or in remission, should consult their physicians regarding the advisability of adding hydrazine sulfate to their present regimens.

This move could be life-sparing or life-saving to you if you have a malignant disease. Regarding this drug's toxicity, since hydrazine sulfate is not a cytotoxic agent (cell-killer), side effects have been characterized as "mild" and frequently transient. Controlled clinical trials have demonstrated no incidence of carcinogenicity or documentation of organ failure as a result of hydrazine sulfate therapy: "There were no significant differences between the protocol arms with regard to myelodepression, gastrointestinal toxicity, renal toxicity, cardiopulmonary toxicity, or neurotoxicity."

Many of you know me as the developer of hydrazine sulfate as an anticancer agent and therefore it would be expected to be in my--"Dr. Gold's"--interest to promote this drug. But it is not Dr. Gold talking. Not Dr. Gold making these recommendations. It is the studies. The controlled clinical trials performed within the confines of the Helsinki Declaration. The controlled clinical trials performed in accordance with internationally accepted scientific principles of experimental biomedical study conduct. Dr. Gold is merely quoting the results of these studies.

These studies in essence suggest that it would be sheer insanity for a cancer patient failing current therapy, not to try hydrazine sulfate. To wait until his/her disease becomes truly terminal, from which there is no return.

But when consulting your doctor, you may hear remarks in good faith such as: "The National Cancer Institute has tested this drug and found it to be ineffective." "This drug's been around a long time. If it were any good, we'd know about it." "This drug is very toxic." "There is no credible evidence that this drug has anticancer activity." Remarks such as these from a trusted medical advisor can serve only to discourage and dissuade you from a try on this drug.

Know, however, there is but one judgment--the controlled clinical trials--that can advise whether a drug trial may be beneficial. The controlled clinical trials properly done--i.e., the Petrov and Harbor-UCLA studies. Your doctor may be unaware of these. Your doctor may be aware of only the incompetently performed National Cancer Institute-sponsored studies, those in violation of the Helsinki Declaration.

You can present your health care provider with copies of the actual Petrov and Harbor-UCLA studies, performed in compliance with the Helsinki Declaration, by visiting the Web site scri.ngen.com and clicking onto "Articles." To the left of each listed article is an icon. By clicking onto the icon, a one-paragraph summary ("abstract") of the published study will appear. By clicking onto the title of the study to the right of the icon, the entire published study will appear. Either the summary or the entire article, as they appear in the medical literature, can be downloaded and then presented to your physician.

Your physician will then have the opportunity to review the pertinent data--the results of properly controlled clinical trials--he/she may not have been previously aware of, and then discuss with you any recommendations as to the appropriateness of hydrazine sulfate as a treatment option for you.

Hydrazine sulfate is presently available by a doctor's prescription filled in a compounding pharmacy. A listing of compounding pharmacies nearest you may be obtained from The International Academy of Compounding Pharmacists, Houston, Texas, 800-927-4227.

As a last word, I know it sounds almost absurd to have a cancer drug that can induce significant anticancer response, largely ignored by the medical establishment and by specific cancer organizations and agencies, such as the National Cancer Institute. But the reality is that the only controlled clinical trials of this drug not in conflict with the internationally ratified Helsinki Declaration--the Petrov and Harbor-UCLA data--say this is the case: That upwards of 50 percent of all cancer patients, even those who are late-stage, can expect an improvement in their cancer status as a result of this treatment.

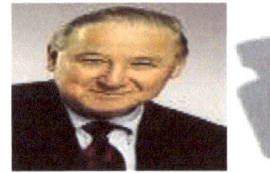 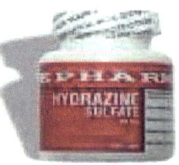

Source: medtruth.blogspot.com Dr. Joseph Gold and HydrazineSulfate, 600 East Genesee Street, Syracuse, NY 13202 Tel: 315-472-6616

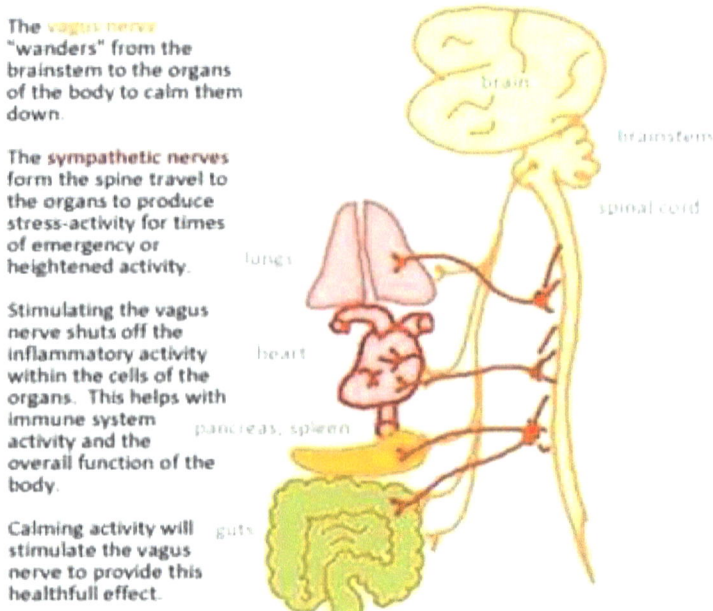

Chanting Divine Names

Toning is the prolonged singing of simple vowel sounds which connects us deeply to our breath and instantly clears our mind. Research has shown that toning and humming stimulate the vagus nerve which can help prevent epileptic seizures, alleviate depression and decrease inflammation. With continued practice, toning, chanting, humming, meditation and Qigong with diaphragmatic breathing will literally "tone" the vagus nerve which can help to regulate the nervous system by slowing the heart rate and lowering blood pressure.

A higher vagal tone index is linked to physical and psychological well-being. A low vagal tone index is linked to inflammation, negative moods, loneliness, and heart attacks. — Psychology Today

Toning is the easiest way for anyone to experience the immediate benefits of sound healing, and the best part is that you don't need anything other than what you've already got — your breath, your voice and your ability to listen.

Chanting is the focused repetition of a word, syllable, mantra or prayer that has the immediate effect of calming our mind. Chanting can be done silently or out loud, and the chant itself can be anything that is meaningful to the chanter. All cultures have a tradition of chanting, from the monasteries of Europe, to the temples of Nepal, to the African savanna, to the sweat lodges and pow-wows of Turtle Island (North America). Chanting divine names like Baha'ullah (Glory of God), Allah'u'Abha (God, the Most Glorious), and the Greatest Name – Ya Baha'u'l-Abha (O Glory of the All-Glorious) can help you connect to this ancient healing practice.

Prayer is conversation with God. God is the great compassionate physician who alone gives true healing.

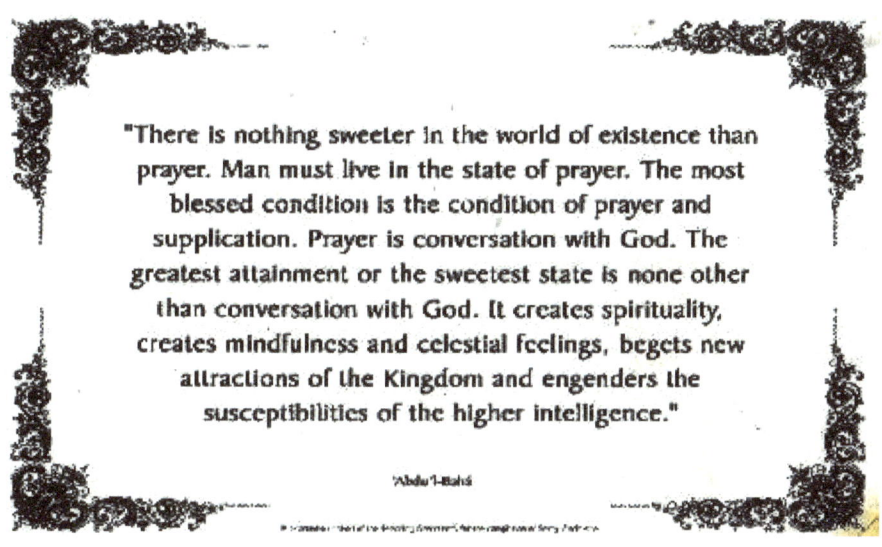

"There is nothing sweeter in the world of existence than prayer. Man must live in the state of prayer. The most blessed condition is the condition of prayer and supplication. Prayer is conversation with God. The greatest attainment or the sweetest state is none other than conversation with God. It creates spirituality, creates mindfulness and celestial feelings, begets new attractions of the Kingdom and engenders the susceptibilities of the higher intelligence."

'Abdu'l-Bahá

Prayer and meditation is like food for the soul or spirit. Praying with prayer beads amplify its effects.

Vagus Nerve Stimulation

Inflammation is the root cause of most chronic diseases and vagus nerve stimulation can effectively reduce inflammation.

Three clinically proven ways to naturally stimulate the vagus nerve are: intracranial intranasal light therapy, auricular therapy and Qi-healing (prana mudra) with Sri Vidya mantra chanting. See Intranasal Light Therapy, page 135

Besides high blood pressure, depression, dementia, migraines, fatigue and anxiety, some people with tinnitus, sleep apnea and epilepsy have been helped with these techniques. Try it! These are life-saving techniques!

The balancing yin yang effect in the body by vagus nerve stimulation activates the Yuan Qi in the central channel not only for healing but also results in samadhi (oneness with Higher Self). Qi is the commander of Blood. Blood is the mother of Qi. Yi (intention) guides Qi. Qi and love are never separate. Hreem Shreem Sauh Hasakaphrem

Why we Should Stimulate the Vagus Nerve in Cancer

Cancer-related fatigue, pain, anxiety, depression, insomnia and cognitive impairment often cooccur in metastatic cancer. Their co-occurrence can be explained by a commonetio logical factor, namely excessive inflammation, which also contributes to tumorigenesis. Recent research shows that the vagus nerve has an anti-inflammatory role and has protective effects against these symptoms and prognosis in various cancers. Initially high vagus nerve activity independently predicts better cancer prognosis, specifically in the metastatic stage, and attenuates these symptoms. Various (semi) experimental studies in humans and animals showed that vagotomy accelerates tumor growth, while vagal nerve activation improves cancer prognosis. Since cancer patients also have a low vagus nerve activity, these points to strong need to activate this nerve and thereby reduce the symptom cluster and prolong survival, via the reduction of inflammation. This article reveals neuro modulation of tumors and proposes a novel adjuvant cancer therapy to improve patients' prognosis and quality of life.

When Shiva and Shakti are reunited, samadhi is the outcome

"Nothing has the greatest power to heal, but Self". The body has the innate power to heal itself, we just need to allow and open up. To be grounded in the Self, to be at home with the Self, to be established in the Self, then the wisdom of the body awakens and guides you. That is the yogic concept of healing.

When the ida and pingala pathways are rebalanced and reunited, and the kundalini shakti in the sushumna (middle channel) is awakened via the vagus nerve Qi-healing with Sri Vidya chanting, samadhi and healing are the outcome.

Thus, it is said in kundalini yoga that when Shiva and Shakti are reunited, samadhi is the resultant outcome. See Subtle Energy System, page 133, Return to Oneness with Shiva

The ida and pingala pathways correspond to the vagus nerve that runs in the left and right side of the neck that connect to the points in the organs down to the abdomen.

The vagus nerve also corresponds to the thrusting channels of the eight extraordinary meridians which can be stimulated by the eight extraordinary meridians Qigong. The large intestine meridian is also connected with the vagus nerve, and by stimulating the points along the meridian by acupuncture and intranasal light therapy can stimulate the vagus nerve.

The other five meridians inside/around nose are: stomach meridian, du meridian, yin-jiao meridian, yang-jiao meridian, and small intestine meridian. These six meridians can be irradiated by Intranasal Light Therapy through multiple nasal reflex.They mediate some of the therapeutic effects of intranasal light therapy. See 8 extraordinary meridians Qigong, page 65, Oneness with Shiva; Guo Lin Qigong, page 55 – Ricardo B Serrano, R.Ac., Originator of Vagus Nerve Qi-healing

After using the Intranasal Light Therapy for 25 minutes, there was a decrease of blood viscosity that can be linked with all of the other major cardiovascular risk factors, including high blood pressure, elevated LDL cholesterol, low HDL, type-II diabetes, metabolic syndrome, obesity, stroke, migraine, dementia, heart attack and cancer. See Intranasal light therapy, page 135

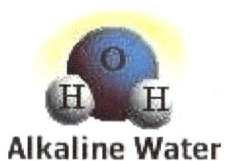

Alkaline Water

What makes the water energized? What is the energy called? The energy is called Prana (Universal life force).

The prana is a vital metaphysical Life force and Light frequency, that exists universally, which underlies all physical actions of the body. It causes the circulation of the blood, movement of cells, and all motions which life of the body depends. It is a force sent forth from the nervous and meridian system by an effort of the will to direct healing.

Prana also is known by different names such as Qi in acupuncture and Traditional Chinese medicine, Ki in Japanese medicine and martial arts, and Shakti in East Indian Yoga or Ayurvedic Medicine.

The individual receives prana, Qi, Ki, or shakti from the sun, food eaten, alkaline or hexagonal kangen water drank, and air breathed. All force or energy received comes from one primal source, and everyone can increase their supply and give it as a "gift" to others through meditation, healing or energizing the water and food eaten. By the act of living spiritually, each receives this gift and therefore can freely share it with others.

"To know the cause of a disease and to understand the use of the various methods by which disease may be prevented amounts to the same thing in effect as being able to cure the malady." – Hippocrates

"Drink alkaline water in order to wash out acidic wastes, universal cause of adult diseases." - Sang Y. Whang

Why Drink Alkaline Water?

1. Ionization (passing an electrical charge through water) raises the pH of tap water from around 6 to 9.5 and increases the anti-oxidants in the water. Ionized water acts as a solvent on acidic waste stored in the body and dissolves it to be removed by the blood.
2. Ionization cuts the size of the water molecular cluster in half. This smaller cluster can penetrate the cellular membranes of the body easier, thus speeding new tissue building and waste removal.
3. Ionization splits the water molecule into H+ and OH- ions. By drinking the water with the alkaline, oxygen rich OH- ions more oxygen is made available to enrich the blood which can increase one's level of energy and promote quicker healing.

4. The ionized OH- molecules have extra electrons that neutralize destructive free radicals circulating throughout the body and thus allow the natural healing processes of the body to predominate and promote health.

These four benefits make ionized water a superior anti-oxidant, that promotes health, as well as anti-aging.

"You're not sick; you're thirsty. Don't treat thirst with medication." - Dr. F. Batmanghelidj, MD

Acid wastes build up in the body in the form of cholesterol, gallstones, kidney stones, arterial plaque, urates, phosphates and sulfates. These acidic waste products are the direct cause of premature aging and the onset of chronic disease.

One of the most cost-effective things you can do for your overall health and well-being is to drink more water and to use a water ionizer to make Alkaline water. Drink alkaline water for health and long life. - Dr. Stefan Kuprowsky, ND

"People who state that alkaline water is snake oil; a water ionizer is a rip-off; acid alkaline theory of disease is nonsense, are dehydrated people who obviously haven't used alkaline water and water ionizer to wash out acidic wastes from their body to experience a better state of health and well-being -- Ricardo B. Serrano, R.Ac.

Alkaline Ionized water closely replicates the natural "living" (electrically charged) qualities of free flowing mountain spring water. It's fresh, delicious, life enhancing water produced right at your own faucet!

Water is the single most important resource for the human body. Water is the most essential nutrient involved in every function of the body. Water accounts for approximately 70% of an individual's complete fat free body mass. In order to function properly, water must be consumed in set quantities in consistent intervals (average of 2.5 liters per day). When not enough water is consumed, people can begin to develop certain illnesses and even accelerate their aging processes.

Now after establishing the importance of water, one must then think what kind of water is good to drink? Many people believe that the water concentrations in coffee, sodas, and energy drinks will be sufficient for the human body to function on optimal levels; but that is incorrect. Simply stated, the water from these beverages is nothing but poor quality distilled water.

Your Answer to Hydration and Better Health Lies in Hexagonal Kangen Water

What is Kangen Water?

Kangen Water - "Return to Origin"

Dating back to its roots in Japan, Kangen Water essentially means "return to origin". Because this beautiful world of ours has been polluted and soiled with human waste, the human body has not been able to reach optimal growth potential. Medical studies have long recognized the devastating effects of high levels of acidity in our bodies. Kangen Water has a pH of 8.5 -11.0 which would then make this water basic or an alkaline. In addition to Kangen waters pH level, tests have also shown a negative ORP (oxidizing reduction potential) rating. Kangen water is perhaps the most effective anti-oxidant and its negative ORP rating further proves that hypothesis. Anti-oxidants can help balance out some of these acids and restore the body to equilibrium or its "original state" as it should be, where we can all grow and flourish.

Free Radicals

Conditions such as exposure to electromagnetic or ultra-violet radiation, alcohol, tobacco, and the stresses that arise in each individual's daily life can all contribute to the build-up of free radicals in one's body. Free radicals are an atomic or molecular species with unpaired electrons on an open shell configuration. The unpaired electrons in these free radicals make it very easy to partake in chemical reactions within the body as it searches to fill its outer most shells with electrons inside of our bodies. Studies have shown that these free radicals account for 70% of all diseases including some forms of cancer, diabetes, and speeding up the aging process. A healthier lifestyle can be achieved immediately as these free radicals are eliminated from our bodies. Kangen Water simply rids these free radicals from our drinking water and bodies through the process of ionization.

Recognizing Alkaline Water

As medical studies have recognized for years, the average human body contains acidity levels that can be harmful to the human body. Alkaline and acidic treatment has been widely used in medical treatments in Japan since the 1960s with success stories of many various illnesses. When patients began requesting medical facilities to continue their treatment in the convenience of their own homes, Enagic Inc. started doing research on how to bring these wondrous machines to the people. After much valuable research, Enagic Inc. of Japan made medical breakthroughs by bringing fortunate people machines that could dispense pure alkaline and acidic water to continue their healthy lifestyles in the comfort of their own homes. To say that this company has been successful in the distribution of these devices would be an understatement in Japan as Enagic Inc. has truly become the top premier water company.

Kangen Water - an antioxidant

It is safe to say that Kangen water is an incredible antioxidant. Some may go as far as to say that Kangen water is more powerful that any single food or vitamin supplement in the world. Simply stated, Kangen water contains active hydrogen which supplies vast amounts of free electrons to our body. This process of electrolysis immediately neutralizes the free radicals in the water and renders it non-poisonous. Most water electrolysis equipment will not create active hydrogen in the water; therefore, the equipment merely produces ionized alkaline water. Because our bodies fluid concentration is roughly two-thirds water, the antioxidant potential of a single glass of Kangen water would be much easier for the body to absorb than expensive vitamin supplements. In fact, instead of breaking down calcium to supply the electrons to neutralize free radicals, Kangen water supplies the active hydrogen to do the job for you. When your body retains the extra calcium that is no longer used to break down free radicals, these calcium minerals can be used to aid in weight loss.

Miracle Healing Water

"Magical miracle healing water" has been found in nature at only a few specific locations throughout the world. These so called "miracle" water sources have been discovered in Mexico, Germany, India, China, Australia, and Japan. Large numbers of people from all over the world wait in line almost every hour of every day to obtain some of this "magical water" at all of these locations. For many years, the healing power of this "magical water" was a mystery, but according, Dr. Sanetaka Shirahata, Graduate School of Genetic Resources Technology, Kyushu University, these so called "miracle waters" all contain active hydrogen in the water. Because active hydrogen has an evaporation rate of 0.3-0.7 seconds after generating it, people had to visit these sources to improve on their chronic illnesses. Hexagonal Kangen water has the same active hydrogen properties and actually improves on this miracle water. With all said and done, Hexagonal Kangen Water can now be produced in the comfort of your own home straight from your tap.

Why Drink Kangen Water?

1. Alkalizes Your Body: Kangen water balances the acidity of the body and makes it real unpleasant for diseases and viruses.
2. Hydrates Your Body: Kangen water transports vitamins, minerals and nutrients at a much faster rate than normal tap water and Kangen water reaches parts of your body that tap water can't get to.
3. Neutralizes Free Radicals: Kangen water is a powerful anti-oxidant; it neutralizes the free radicals in your body.
4. Cleans the Colon and Eliminates the Root of Sickness: Kangen water cleanses your colon which may include poisoning fecal matter from days, weeks, months, or even years!

5. Alkaline/Ionized Water: Has been known to help treat constipation, diabetes, dry skin, high blood pressure, indigestion, obesity, osteoporosis, tension headaches and other ailments.

Dr. Zoltan P. Rona's article Why Purified Water is Bad for You has personally opened my eyes to realize that my symptoms such as heartburn, digestive disorder, high blood pressure, eye problem, hair loss, hypothyroidism, tooth loss and other body pain symptoms are mainly caused by drinking *distilled water* for seven years. These symptoms have disappeared by not drinking purified acidic distilled and RO (reverse-osmosis) water, and drinking alkaline ionized water, instead.

I have been drinking alkaline ionized water (Kangen water) for 6 years now together with other preventative health measures to maintain my health, and have recommended drinking kangen alkaline ionized water to my clients with various disease symptoms who have greatly benefited from its home use together with practicing Qigong and meditation, eating a balanced diet, taking tonic herbs, and exercising outside to get fresh air and sunlight.

I might add that drinking commercially bottled water is as bad as drinking purified water because most bottled water is either purified through distillation and reverse osmosis that produces acidic water which contributes to acidosis and oxidation caused diseases. So what does this leave most number of people who want to drink alkaline ionized water (Kangen water)? The most obvious alternative is to have your own Kangen alkaline water ionizer machine.

Of course, choosing the right Kangen alkaline water ionizer machine to obtain alkaline ionized water that will optimally correct the acid/alkaline balance, and have hydrating and anti-oxidant properties in the body, is important. I will gladly assist my interested clients in answering inquiries, in choosing the right Enagic Kangen water ionizer machine for home use, and in instructing in its proper use to obtain maximum health benefits. As an Enagic Distributor ID # 1244382, please contact me by email at kangen@qigonghealer.com and calling 604-987-1797 to make an appointment and get a free gallon of hexagonal kangen water. Thank you!

Throughout our lives, we exist mostly as water. This connection to water applies to everyone, all over the world. So how can people live happy and healthy lives? The answer is to purify the water that makes up your body. Water in a river remains pure because it is moving. When water becomes trapped, it dies. Therefore, water must constantly be circulated. The water - or blood - in the bodies of the sick is usually stagnant. When blood stops flowing, the body starts to decay, and if the blood in your brain stops, it can be life threatening. We all have an important mission: To make water clear again, and to create a world that is easy and healthy to live in. In order to accomplish our mission, we must first make sure that our hearts are clear and unpolluted. If all the people of the world can have love and gratitude, the pristine beauty of the earth will once again return.

"I believe that prior to Adam and Eve water itself held the consciousness of God -- that God's intention was put into the medium of water, and that this was used in the creation of Earth and Nature. In other words, all of the information needed for God's Creation was reflected in the water.

And then we -- Adam and Eve -- were placed on Earth to be the caretakers for this Creation of God. I believe that water held the consciousness of God until then, but that after the caretakers were placed on Earth, water became an empty vessel to mirror and reflect what was in the heart. It became a container to carry energy and information. Therefore, since this time, I think water has taken on the quality of simply reflecting the energies and thoughts that it is exposed to; that it no longer has its own consciousness. Water reflects the consciousness of the human race." - Masaro Emoto, The Hidden Messages of Water

Proper Breathing

As important as the kind of water you drink is the way you breathe for energy and healing during meditation. Of course, the quality of air you breathe is also very important that is unpolluted, very close to lakes, rivers, seashore and trees where there are plenty of negative ions (see Negative Ion Therapy, page 108) especially in the early morning hours of the day.

Proper breathing may reduce the risk of cancer, since cancer cells are the only cells that do not like oxygen.

Dr. Otto Warburg won the Nobel Prize in Medicine in 1931 for this discovery, and oxygenation treatments have been used to kill cancer cells as a result. Conversely, depriving cells of oxygen is thought to increase the likelihood of their turning cancerous.

Low oxygen levels in the body also encourage acid conditions, increasing the risk of disease, including cancer, whereas good breathing will encourage alkalinity and therefore good health.

Dr. Warburg has made it clear that the root cause of cancer is oxygen deficiency, which creates an acidic state in the human body. Dr. Warburg also discovered that cancer cells are anaerobic (do not breathe oxygen) and cannot survive in the presence of high levels of oxygen, as found in an alkaline state.

Dr. Warburg was director of the Kaiser Wilhelm Institute (now Max Planck Institute) for cell physiology at Berlin. He investigated the mutation of tumours and the respiration of cells, particularly cancer cells.

Therapeutic Diaphragmatic Breathing

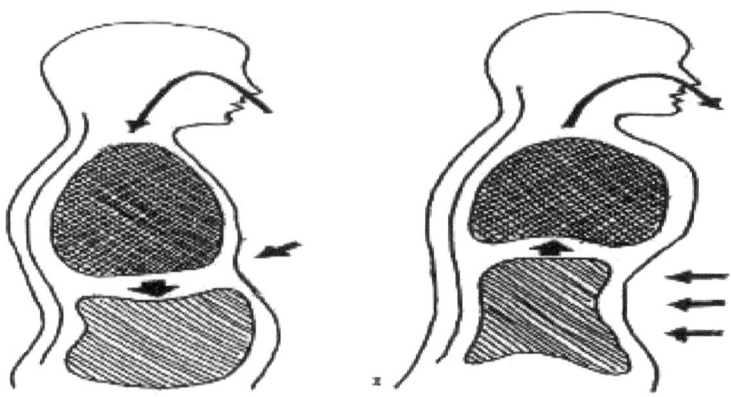

"Breathing is the most important part of the GuoLin Qigong practice and other Qigong forms."

– Ricardo B Serrano, R.Ac.

Walking Qigong incorporates therapeutic diaphragmatic breathing (**XiXi Hu).** By walking with the hands and feet moving in proper gestures, and co-ordinating with rhythmic breathing (inhaling twice and exhaling once), practitioners absorb a large quantity of oxygen so that their meridians can be regulated, flow of qi and blood can be stimulated, and their body and mind can be nourished by the nature. Thousands of practitioners suffering from medium or late stage of cancers, or chronic diseases have been cured by consistently practicing Guo Lin Qigong.

Diaphragmatic breathing is also done with the tip of tongue touching the upper palate in the Standing Qigong incorporated with Walking Qigong.

For more info on Guo Lin Qigong, read How Guo Lin Qigong works? page 55; What is Guo Lin Qigong? page 68; Get Well Verse for Cancer patients, page 112; and Introduction to Guo Lin Qigong, page 120.

"Cancerous tissues are acidic, whereas healthy tissues are alkaline. Water splits into H+ and OH- ions, if there is an excess of H+ ions, it is acidic; if there is an excess of OH- ions, then it is alkaline." - Dr. Otto Warburg

In his work "The Metabolism of Tumours," Warburg demonstrated that "all forms of cancer are characterized by two basic conditions: acidosis and hypoxia (lack of oxygen). Lack of oxygen and acidosis are two sides of the same coin: where you have one, you have the other." "All normal cells have an absolute requirement for oxygen, but cancer cells can live without oxygen – a rule without exception. Deprive a cell 35% of its oxygen for 48 hours and it may become cancerous."

Source: The Prime Cause of Cancer, Dr. Otto Warburg Lecture delivered to Nobel Laureates, June 30, 1966 at Lindau, Lake Constance, Germany.

The true cause of cancer

Herman Aihara, in his book entitled "Acid & Alkaline", states that: "If the condition of our extra cellular fluids, especially the blood, becomes acidic, our physical condition will first manifest tiredness, proneness to catching colds, etc. When these fluids become more acidic, our condition then manifests pains and suffering such as headaches, chest pains, stomach aches, etc. According to Keiichi Morishita in his *Hidden Truth of Cancer*, if the blood develops a more acidic condition, then our body inevitably deposits these excess acidic substances in some area of the body such so that the blood will be able to maintain an alkaline condition.

As this this tendency continues, such areas increase in acidity and some cells die; then these dead cells themselves turn into acids. However, some other cells may adapt in that environment. In other words, instead of dying - as normal cells do in an acid environment - some cells survive by becoming abnormal cells. These abnormal cells are called malignant cells. Malignant cells do not correspond with brain function nor with our own DNA memory code. Therefore, malignant cells grow indefinitely and without order. This is cancer.

Modern medicine in America treats these malignant cells as if they were bacteria or viruses. It uses chemotherapy, radiation, and surgery to treat cancer. Yet none of these treatments will help very much, if after all of that, the acidic environment remains.

Drinking water that has a high alkaline pH, because of its de-acidifying effect, will help in preventing cancer. In Asia, alkaline water is regularly served to patients, and is considered a regular part of treatment."

Mr. Aihara does not mention anything about the lack of oxygen but rather talks about the acidification of extra cellular fluids which causes cancer. Dr. Warburg states that the primary cause of cancer is the lack of oxygen in a cell, like a plant cell. He didn't know what caused the lack of oxygen.

Dr. Warburg was dealing with the symptoms of acid build ups rather than the cause. Mr. Aihara was hitting the nail right on the head. For this reason, the German solution is to alleviate the symptoms, that is, to supply more oxygen, while the Japanese solution is to reduce the acidity, the very cause, by alkaline diet and / or alkaline water.

Qi is life-force that animates the forms of the world. It is the vibratory nature of life phenomena – the flow that is happening continuously at molecular, atomic and sub-atomic levels. In Japan it is called "ki," and in India, "prana" or "shakti." The ancient Egyptians referred to it as "ka," and the ancient Greeks as "pneuma." For Native Americans it is the "Great Spirit" and for Christians, the "Holy Spirit." In Africa it's known as "ashe" and in Hawaii as "ha" or "mana." Wilhelm Reich also called it as orgone, negative ions or negative entropy.

Most ailments especially cancer and kidney diseases are the result of an imbalance in the body's electrical Wei Qi field, usually due to a drop in supply of anions or negatively charged ions. Guo Lin Qigong and electromagnetic healing therapy can replenish the negative ions needed for healing cancer and chronic diseases. See Electrotherapy, page 103 and Negative Ion Therapy, page 108

To provide alkaline ionized water is to preserve men's health

To love is to provide, and to provide is to preserve.

God provides pure natural water to preserve men's health.

Men has polluted water and made it acidic making tap water unfit to drink.

God inspired men to filter and ionize tap water to return water to its origin and make water fit to drink, once more.

To provide alkaline ionized water via water ionizer from tap water making it pure natural water for drinking is to preserve men's health.

How does alkaline water preserve health? Drinking alkaline ionized water neutralizes and washes out acidic wastes, the root cause of men's diseases, and restores the acid (yang) and alkaline (yin) balance preserving men's health and long life. To love is to provide, and to provide is to preserve. – Ricardo B Serrano, R.Ac.

How Guo Lin Qigong works

Guo Lin Qi Gong works by keeping the energy strong to help the immune system, maximising our own organs' powerful ability to help deal with illness and cancers.

1. Breathing and walking – two breaths in, one breath out maximises the body's ability to carry oxygen to kill cancer cells.

2. Adjusting the channels to tonify (enrich) the blood and energy for a stronger immune system. Guo Lin Qi Gong adjusts the bio-electric current to help kill the cancer cells.

3. Guo Lin Qi Gong is like a walking meditation, helping to relax, reduce anxiety and maintain a positive and balanced inner environment.

Guo Lin Qi Gong helps ease the side effects of medical treatment and promotes better sleep and a healthier appetite.

For more info on Guo Lin Qigong, read What is Guo Lin Qigong? page 68; Get Well Verse for Cancer patients, page 112; and Introduction to Guo Lin Qigong, page 120.

Guolin New Qigong adopts 3 principles in healing cancer:

1. Increasing Oxygenation

2. Improving Circulation

3. Stabilizing Emotions

Traditional Chinese medicine holds that disease occurs when there is stagnation of qi which will be cured when the circulation of qi and blood is improved. Hence, with proper execution of Relaxation (sung jing), Concentration (yi lian) and Breathing (hu xi) in qigong exercises, one will be able to achieve the 3 fundamental principles mentioned above advocated by Guolin in activating the flow of qi (vital life energy). One will be able to sleep well, eat well, and strengthen the immune system to heal even the most chronic diseases.

It is also acknowledged in the western medicine that cancer cells can be suppressed when oxygen level is increased to eight times more than ordinary. The Guolin double inhalations (xi xi) in the Walking Qigong exercise increases the oxygen in-take 20 times more than the normal that causes the retardation of cancer cells growth

There are 5 basic therapies a cancer patient can adhere to in order to fight cancer:

1. Western Therapy: Surgery, Radiotherapy or Chemotherapy

2. Chinese Therapy: Acupuncture or Chinese Medicine

3. Change Lifestyles

4. Diet

5. Guolin Qigong

Note: Madam Guo Lin introduced 3-prongs approach, however with the Stress of modern living and environment, we have included no. 3 & 4

To allow readers a better perspective, attached herewith the excerpt from a former President Dr Amir Farid Dato Isahak:

The most important exercise in Guolin Qigong is the walking exercises whereby the breathing, footstep and body and arm movements are consciously coordinated to energize the body. It is this exercise that has benefited chronic disease patients most. This qigong-walk doubles or even triples one's walking distance in terms of endurance and stamina compared with ordinary walking.

Those who are ill or receiving hazardous cancer treatments will find their ability to cope with the illness or the side-effects of the treatment much better. Those who are unable to walk can do stationary exercises first. But it is always better to have a preventive attitude than to wait for illness to strike before learning qigong.

Dr Amir Farid bin Dato Isahak, President (Former), Guolin Qigong Association Malaysia

Testimonials:

1. Peter Kwok - 59 years old (11 years)

Peter Kwok has survived kidney cancer for 11 years.

2. Master Ho Peng - 85 years old (30 years)

Master Ho Peng, 85 years old, was the founder of Persatuan Guolin Qigong Malaysia. He was inflicted with rectal cancer in 1982 but successfully cured himself from cancer by just practising Guolin Qigong.

3. Wong Peng Yem - 72 years old (29 years)

Wong Peng Yem has survived fourth stage colon cancer for 29 years. He had the disease in 1983 and a recurrence in 2003.

4. Maggie Chen - 43 years old (12 years)

Maggie is a fouth stage cancer survivor. She had Hodgkin's Lymphoma 12 years ago. Currently she is a Guolin Qigong Station Master.

5. Wong Sui Nyun - 53 years old (5 years)

Wong Sui Nyun was inflicted with breast cancer in 2007 and had four surgeries in two years

6. Angie Ng - 58 years old (6 years)

Angie says that cancer patients and survivors should take note of sleep, diet, exercise and mood.

7. Yu Da Yuan, Chairman of the Beijing Anti-Cancer Assoc. (22-year Cancer survivor), Zhang Ji, (8-year Breast Cancer survivor), Sun Cai Yun, Secretary of the Beijing Anti-Cancer Association. (20-year Breast Cancer Survivor). These testimonials dated July, 2000.

For more info on Guo Lin Qigong, read What is Guo Lin Qigong? page 68; Get Well Verse for Cancer patients, page 112; and Introduction to Guo Lin Qigong, page 120.

Cessiac & Yuccalive

These North American native Indian herbal remedies were introduced into China, the herbal kingdom, in 1993. There were several ingredients in the remedies that even the Chinese did not have any information on them. At the requirement of the Ministry of Health of China, numerous tests and studies were conducted by three major hospitals in China. These hospitals included the Beijing Chinese Medicine University East Gate Hospital, the People's Hospital of Guangdong Province, and the Guangzhou City Cancer Hospital. The tests and studies included medicinal test, toxicity test, immunological test, tumor inhibition test, and a 245 cases clinical study. Import permits were finally granted in 1996 by the Ministry of Health of China for these two herbal formulas to be imported into China as the first ever non-traditional Chinese medicine for a Class A disease. The reports here show the results of the tests and studies done in China. It was based on these results that the effectiveness of these herbal formulas were confirmed and the import permits were granted

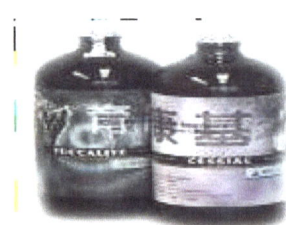

Imported from Canada, "C" Formula and "Y" Formula are oral liquid medicine extracted from pure natural plants and have been used abroad, especially in North America, for seventy years. The preliminary clinical studies in China have shown that the combined use of the two drugs has favorable therapeutical effect on tumor and various diseases resulting from immunologic deficiency. To provide laboratory evidence for further promotion of the two drugs on clinical use, we studied the tumor-inhibition effect of the combined use of the two drugs on mice contracted with cancer. This study was conducted according to the "Guidelines on Pre-clinical Study of New Chinese Medicine", Ministry of Health of China, 1993.

Acute Toxicity test through oral administration on mouse: select 30 mice weight between 20 to 22g. 15 MALE AND 15 FEMALE. Feed mice with the entire dosage condensed Formula - (equivalent to the strength of 70.61 ml/kg. of the original medicine). Observe mice for 7 days after feeding. All mice survived with a normal appetite. It is observed that the mice can take up to 70.61 ml./kg. of "Y" Formula orally without any problem. (For an average adult of 50 kg. in China, normal dosage is 30 ml. per day orally.) The dosage in this test is equivalent to 117 times of the normal dosage. The dosage of 20 ml. per day per adult is recommended for clinical testing.

It is concluded that oral administration of the "Y" Formula is safe.

Cause of Cancer and other Chronic Immune Dysfunction Syndromes

The main cause of cancer and other chronic immune (Wei) dysfunction syndromes is a weakened or suppressed immune system (Wei Qi) due to many causative factors which can be categorized into climatic changes, food factors, emotional factors and hereditary factors.

Climatic Changes and External Factors

According to Chinese medical theory, dampness or humidity weakens the energy of the spleen-pancreas complex aggravating any immuno-suppressed condition. The continuous air pollution, indiscriminate use of artificial chemicals, disrespectful dumping of tons of garbage into our rivers and seas, and the creation of holes in the ozone layer. Burning of forests has increased the CO2 in our atmosphere causing an increase in temperature enough to flood coastal cities and create dryness in productive farmlands, and deplete our supply of vital oxygen.

Another of the external factors is the overuse of medications presently killing more people a year than car accidents. Antibiotics have become a home remedy for anything that looks like an innocent cold, killing friendly bacteria in our gut and allowing yeast overgrowth in increasing numbers. The "pill" once hailed as sexual liberation, has so many side effects (yeast overgrowth one of them) that it is incredible to me that so many women are still taking it. And of course, cortisone, radiation therapy, anti-cancer drugs all suppress the very immune system they are supposed to support!

Food Factors and Changes

We have processed the goodness out of our foods, ingested toxic metals from our cooking methods, increased the fat intake, decreased the dietary fiber with chronic constipation and degenerative diseases as a consequence. But the biggest threat to our health is the enormous intake of sugar and aspartame (Nutrasweet, Sweet 'N Low). There is also consistent evidence of contaminated poultry and injection of antibiotics and hormones into meat. So what does the American public think? Are they just going to eat this meat anyway? I guess they are. But don't try to sell me the idea that we have the best food in the world. Is it not ironic that we have a special "health food" section? What shall we call those other foods? "Unhealthy foods"? You know, we should.

Emotions

Eastern medicine recognized the relationship between emotions and the damage they do to organs 5,000 years ago. You can easily guess which one damages the immune system (Wei Qi) raising the rate of "wear and tear" within the body. Yes, it is worry, STRESS. Blame whatever you will -- job, spouse, bills, kids, the complexity of life -- stress has become one of America's most common health problems. In every cancer, Chronic Fatigue Syndrome and other CIDS patient that I have seen in my practice, stress was the ultimate triggering factor, the straw that broke the camel's back. And most often, it is the single cause of relapse. Only very recently has Western medicine begun investigating stress.

Hereditary Factors

Heredity is one of the main means of spreading CIDS. The biggest culprit here is the yeast cell, Candida albicans. Candida is considered the number one aggressor when our immune system is suppressed. With the increased progesterone in the third trimester of pregnancy, CIDS patients with Candida see an aggravation to their condition. Unrecognized (mistake #1) or insufficiently treated by doctors (mistake #2), yeast cells are transmitted to the newborn who may be born with thrush, but more likely will start showing symptoms of ear infections. And since Candida collects fluid in the middle ear, pressing against the ear drum, imitating a bacterial infection, antibiotics are given in repetitive doses (mistake #3), providing the ideal climate to enhance the growth of the yeast cell. It is not uncommon to see 4 year-olds who have been on antibiotics for almost all of their short lives. The rest is a modern classic. These children crave sugar, become hyperactive, receive Ritalin, demonstrate learning disabilities and are labelled problems (Mistakes innumerable). Those children never get a chance! CIDS is NOT a disease of "Yuppies"; it affects children and adolescents in much greater numbers than you suspect.

Knowing that the above factors are the causes of a suppressed system and secondarily lead to an invasion of yeast, viruses, bacteria and parasites, we realize that although the problem cannot be rectified by a single medication (which is only a dream), it can be controlled by a total holistic approach.

Signs of a Depressed Immune System

The very first micro-organism to sense the decreased strength of our immune system (Wei Qi) is the Candida cell. In fact it starts multiplying before the patient exhibits one single symptom. Hence, immuno-suppressed patients present themselves with yeast symptoms. Of course, the reader thinks about a vaginal yeast infection, and indeed, millions of victims show such a symptom. Alas, this is not all. Multiple food sensitivities, bloating, gas, constipation or loose bowels, PMS, no menstrual cycle at all, cravings for sugar and carbohydrates, inability to lose weight, loss of short-term memory and concentration, panic attacks, inability to hold chiropractic adjustments, dizzy spells, postnasal drip, mood swings, urination frequency and burning, loss of sexual desire, metallic taste in the mouth and irritability, all are symptoms of yeast overgrowth. Once the patient's immune system is busy fighting this massive yeast invasion, viruses such as Herpes Simplex family (like CEBV) have an easy time multiplying and exhibiting their own symptomatology -- muscle fatigue, sore throats, flu-like symptoms, low grade fevers and enlarged cervical lymph nodes. Often a hypersensitivity towards sunlight and sound is noted. The patient catches one cold after another, sensitivities towards the environment increase, and the patient feels like he will never recover from an endless flu. As if he does not have enough to deal with already, almost every CIDS is invaded by the ultimate enemy, parasites. They will add their own ailments (loose stools, ravenous appetite with weight loss) but often blend symptoms with those of yeast and viruses.

Therapeutic Measures

Avoid greasy and fatty foods. Shun the number one killer, sugar (fructose, sucrose, corn syrup, honey). I have already mentioned to avoid aspartame at all costs. The diet of an immuno-suppressed patient should be a high protein, low carbohydrate alkaline one. Avoid breads, dairy products (except butter and eggs), vinegar, apples, pears, grapes, mushrooms, canned foods, coffee, wine, beer, champagne or anything else that is fermented (miso and tofu). Every CIDS patient would show 50% improvement simply by following these guidelines.

Emotional stress factors should be faced and handled through talk therapy with a friend or counsellor (should be a good listener).

Acupuncture is another Chinese therapeutic method besides Qigong for changing the flow or quality of Qi or life force and rebalancing body energies. It has been used to treat persistent pain, arthritis, asthma, infertility, and acute and chronic diseases. In cancer, it can alleviate pain and functional disorders associated with the illness, for example, improving the ability to swallow in victims of esophageal cancer. Acupuncture is also used to mitigate the side effects of chemotherapy and radiation, and has been employed as a primary treatment for early signs of breast and cervical cancer, though the Chinese are more likely to utilize herbal remedies to support immunity and control malignant growth. Acupuncture can also be helpful in stress reduction and the alleviation of pain.

Leukemia has been successfully treated with acupuncture therapy. In addition, acupuncture has exhibited a wide range of actions in boosting immunity, including increasing the number of white blood cells, boosting natural killer cell activity, and increasing the amount of B-cells, which manufacture antibodies, chemicals that help destroy foreign invaders in the body. Acupuncture also elevates the levels of circulating immunoglobulins and stimulates the production of red blood cells.

Learning how to breathe (see Guolin Qigong, page 53) and how to meditate such as the Merkaba meditation or Holographic Sound Healing will greatly magnify the spiritual healing techniques the patient is having and heal holographically increasing the patient's Wei Qi (vital energy) a thousand fold, opening one's heart to unconditional love and activating the light body (Merkaba) of the patient.

The two herbal formulas which are time tested and scientifically proven and improved in mainland China to detoxify the blood, cells and detox organs (such as the liver, bowels, kidney and lungs) are "C" Cessiac and "Y" Yuccalive and which consequently build and strengthen the immune system (Wei Qi).

Obviously, we have to increase the strength of our immune system (Wei-Yong Qi), and this can be achieved through numerous possible treatments. Qigong, Alkaline Kangen Water, sun gazing, acupuncture, moxibustion, pranic healing, resveratrol, germanium, coenzyme Q10, Vitamin C, Beta carotene, Antioxidant (grapeseed, bilberry, cranberry extract), Horsetail Grass extract, Milk Thistle, Green tea, Pau d'arco, Chaparral, Astragalus, Echinacea, Guyabano, Sun Chlorella (Seaweed Extract), Reishi mushroom, Turmeric (*Curcumin*), Buteyko breathing, garlic, Ozone therapy, Vitamin E, Zinc, Green drinks, Virgin Coconut Oil, Microflora (Super-Neoflora) containing a specific bacteria, Bacillus Latersporus, exercise and are just a few that can be tried. By effectively treating the underlying causes of the suppression of the immune system by yeast, parasites, viruses and bacteria, and by avoiding the triggering factors mentioned, one will allow the immune system to restore itself. More than ever in this world, this is a must. If you are not going to start today, when will you start? And if you don't do it for yourself, who will?

Dr. Mirko Beljanski's work expounded by Dr. Morton Walker's book "Cancer's Cause, Cancer's Cure" showed the environmental effects of pollution on the DNA of cells which contribute to tumorgenesis and can be healed through the use of botanical extracts of *Rauwolfia vomitoria* and *Pao Pereira, Ginkgo Biloba* with *RNA fragments* . See beljanski.com and natural-source.com

References:

- Peak Immunity by Dr. Luc De Schepper, MD, PhD, LAc
- Maximum Immunity by Michael A. Weiner, PhD
- Understanding Your Immune System by Eve Potts and Marion Morra
- The Yeast Syndrome by John Trowbridge, MD and Morton Walker, DPM
- Candida, The Symptoms, The Causes, The Cure by Luc De Schepper, MD, DAc
- Eating Alive, Prevention thru Good Nutrition by John Matsen, ND
- Oxygen Therapies, A New Way of Approaching Disease by Ed McCabe
- Oxygen Healing Therapies by Nathaniel Altman
- Alternative Medicine, the Definitive Guide by Burton Goldberg Group
- Healing with Whole Foods by Paul Pitchford
- Advanced Pranic Healing by Master Choa Kok Sui
- The Canary and Chronic Fatigue by Majid Ali, MD
- Options, the Alternative Cancer Therapy Book by Richard Walters
- The New Nutrition, Medicine for the Millenium by Michael Colgan, PhD
- The Immune System Cure by Lorna VanderHaeghe & Patrick Bouic, PhD
- Cancer's Cause, Cancer's Cure by Dr. Morton Walker, DPM
- Anti Cancer: A New Way of Life by Dr. David Servan-Schreiber, MD, 2008.

How and why garlic works At present, it is generally considered by most researchers that the sulfur-containing compounds in garlic, especially allicin, alliin, cycroalliin, and diallyldisulphide - there are 33 such compounds isolated as of now - are the most active substances.

Reference: The Miracle of Garlic by Paavo Airola, 1978, pages 22-23, 32-35

At present, research and clinical observations quoted previously have shown the following active factors being present in garlic (Allium Sativum):

- **Allicin**, the substance in garlic that is believed to be largely responsible for garlic's antibacterial and anti-inflammatory effects. Allicin is also the odorous factor in garlic.
- **Alliin**, a sulfur-containing amino acid in garlic from which allicin is made by the action of the enzyme alliinase. Russian studies ascribed the antibiotic effect on garlic to its alliin content.
- **Diallyldisulphide-oxide**, a chemical compound into which allicin is changed in the system. The essential oil of garlic contains 6% allylpropyldisulphide and 60% diallyldisulphide. The cholesterol and lipid-lowering effect of garlic is attributed to the presence of this factor.
- **Gurwitch rays**, the mitogenetic radiation factor that stimulates cell growth and has a rejuvenating stimulating effect on all body functions.
- **Anti-hemolytic** factor, responsible for its beneficial effect in the treatment of anemia. Note: this factor was proven to be present only in allicin-free garlic preparations, such as Kyolic or Leopin.
- **Anti-arthritic** factor, as shown in Japanese studies at Fukuyama Hospital
- **Sugar-regulating** factor, which makes garlic useful as an adjunct in the treatment of both diabetes and hypoglycemia.
- **Antioxidant** factor. Garlic was shown to inhibit peroxidation (rancidity) of foods, and thus, can be used as a natural preservative.
- **Anti-coagulant** factor. According to clinical studies, garlic contains effective anti-coagulant factors.
- **Anti-tumor factor.** Garlic has a high content of germanium that has cancer preventive and curative effect.
- **Allithiamine**. Garlic is an excellent source of biologically active compounds of vitamin B1. Japanese researchers (Matsukawa et al.) have isolated from garlic a substance, allithiamine, which is formed by the action of vitamin B1 on alliin. This component has been found to have beneficial therapeutic properties and to be effective, among other things, in preventing and curing beriberi.
- **Selenium**. Garlic is also an excellent source of biologically active selenium, and it is believed that garlic's anti-atherosclerotic property (preventing platelet adhesion and clot formation) is due to its high selenium content. Selenium also normalizes blood pressure and has been shown to protect against infections.

The mineral content of garlic, on the other hand, is considerable. Garlic contains manganese, copper, iron, zinc, sulfur, calcium, aluminum, chlorine, germanium, and selenium. The sulfur content of garlic is one of the highest of all vegetables. The selenium content is most remarkable - in fact, garlic is the best known natural source of selenium. On a wet basis, garlic contains 9.3 γ/100 g. of selenium, which is 0.44 p.p.m on a dry weight basis. Selenium is becoming more and more recognized as one of the most important trace elements in human nutrition. Garlic's antioxidant activity is probably due to its selenium content, since selenium is a strong antioxidant; its biological activity is closely related to vitamin E. Selenium may slow down aging processes by an inhibiting action on the formation of free radicals. This may explain why most of the centenarians whom I studied in Bulgaria and Russia are heavy garlic consumers. Selenium also can protect from toxic damage caused by mercury poisoning. As you can see, many of the best-known properties of garlic, such as antioxidant, anti-aging, and anti-toxin activity, may simply be due to its rich content of the miracle-working mineral, selenium. Brewer's yeast is another good source of selenium.

Here is a partial list of ailments that have been successfully treated by raw garlic or garlic extracts: high blood pressure, atherosclerosis, tuberculosis, diabetes, arthritis, cancer, hypoglycemia, bronchits, asthma (garlic juice mixed with comfrey juice), whooping cough, pneumonia, common cold, allergies, intestinal worms, intestinal putrefaction and gas, parasitic diarrhea, dysentery, insomnia

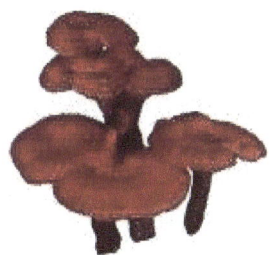

Reishi Mushroom

The Reishi mushroom, also known by its formal name of Ganoderma and its Chinese name Ling Zhi, has attained an unparalleled reputation in the Orient as the ultimate herbal substance. For over three thousand years it has been the most sought-after product of nature by mountain sages and by the emperors and empresses of all Eastern nations. In the first Chinese herbal text (Shen Nong's Pharmacopeia) written about 2400 years ago, Reishi was classified as a "superior herb" which is defined as one that "serves to maintain life, promote radiant health and long life because of its normalizing action, and to cause no side effects, even when used continuously." That ancient book said that "continuous consumption of Reishi makes your body light and young, lengthens your life and turns you into one like the immortal who never dies." Thus Reishi was traditionally called "the mushroom of immortality."

The Reishi Mushroom grows wild only upon old trees and roots of certain types of trees in remote mountain forests of China, Japan and Korea. Only in the fifteen years have we seen the cultivation of Reishi, and thus the commercial availability of this amazing health product. Reishi has been the object of intensive scientific studies to discern its many health functions from a modern perspective. Traditionally, Reishi is believed to be a tonic to all of the body's energies. It was revered as a major tonic to each of the three Treasures, Jing, Qi and Shen.

As a Jing (Essence) tonic, Reishi is believed to have major life lengthening effects when consumed over a long period of time. It is believed to build primal power and to replenish energy spent handling stressful situations.

As a Qi (Vitality) tonic, Reishi is used to build energy, although it is slightly sedative in the short run. It is most famous as an herb used to build the immune system. Many studies done in Japan have shown Reishi to have a powerful effect on the body's overall resistance to disease. Reishi is believed by Japanese and Chinese researchers to have a regulatory effect on the immune system, bringing up immune functions in cases of immunodeficiency and reducing the excesses associated with auto-immune conditions. Reishi is a superb tonic for people who suffer from chronic allergies. Reishi is also believed to have major benefits on the lungs and liver. Studies done in Japan have shown that Reishi protects the liver from damage due to toxic chemicals, including pharmaceutical metabolites. Furthermore, studies done in Japan and elsewhere have also demonstrated that Reishi is beneficial to the cardiovascular system, since it appears to help regulate coronary and cerebral blood flow and also seems to help reduce levels of blood lipids and in lowering elevated cholesterol.

As a Shen (Spirit) tonic, nothing compares to Reishi. It is simply the greatest Shen tonic of them all. It is believed by the Chinese to protect the Spirit and to nurture the growth of intelligence, wisdom and spiritual insight. Reishi is a superb anti-stress herb. Everyone who takes Reishi notices the peacefulness that seems to accompany its use. Many people are able to stop using chemical drugs. And Reishi seems to be cumulative, gradually strengthening the nerves and actually changing how we perceive life. It has routinely been used by mountain hermits, monks, Daoist adepts and spiritual seekers throughout Asia because it was believed to help calm the mind, ease tension, strengthen the nerves, improve memory, sharpen concentration and focus, build will power and, as a result, help build wisdom. That is why it was called the "Mushroom of Spiritual Potency" by these seekers. The people of Asia believe more than ever in Reishi's power to improve the quality of life by improving the inner life of a human being. All the scientific validation only explains the physical nature of Reishi, but it is the profound ability of Reishi to improve one's life on every plane that makes it so incredible.

Studies done in Asia indicate that Reishi is a supreme health food supplement that has virtually no toxicity or side effects.

There are many Reishi products coming to the market at this time, but very few are truly excellent. Reishi must be extracted to be digestible and assimilable. Unfortunately, most Reishi products are not extracted and most are made from inferior quality hot house mushrooms or use inferior cultivated Ganoderma mycelium.
Other Common Names: Reishi mushroom, Ling Zhi, Ganoderma

Pharmaceutical Latin: Ganoderma

Pinyin: Ling Zhi

Treasures: Jing, Qi and Shen

Atmospheric Energy: Neutral or slightly warm

Organ Meridian Systems: Heart, Liver, Lungs, Kidney

Part Used and Form: Fruiting body, spores, mycelium

Primary Functions; Nourishing tonic, tonic to the three treasures (Jing, Qi and Shen), builds body resistance, detoxifying, aphrodisiac, sedative, prolongs life and enhances intelligence and wisdom.

Qualities

Ganoderma is arguably the most revered herbal substance in Asia, certainly ranking with ginseng as the elite substance for the attainment of radiant health, longevity and spiritual attainment. It has maintained that position for at least 2000 years, and its reputation and value are only increasing. Numerous legends provide a rich and extensive record of Ganoderma in Asian society.

Reishi has traditionally been used as an anti-aging herb and has been used for many diseases and disorders as well. It has long been a favorite tonic food supplement by the Chinese Royal family and virtually anyone who could obtain it. Ganoderma was particularly revered by the followers of the Taoist tradition as the "Elixir of Immortality." Taoists have continuously claimed that Reishi promotes calmness, centeredness, balance, inner awareness and inner strength. They have used it to improve meditative practices and to protect the body, mind and spirit so that the adept could attain both a long and healthy life and spiritual immortality. Due to its rarity, the common people could rarely obtain a Reishi mushroom, but it was popularly revered as a greater treasure than any jewel.

Since Reishi has been known to have many functions, it has been the subject of a great deal of research in recent years. It is absolutely safe, being non-toxic. It ranks in Asia with Ginseng, Deer Antler, Astragalus and Cordyceps as a pre-eminent tool in the attainment of radiant health.

Its health benefits of Reishi are extremely broad and it is virtually non-toxic. Though it is now used much like ginseng, Eleutherococcus and Astragalus as a general tonic to help develop energy, to improve digestion and to improve sleep, scientists are exploring its potential in their terms.

Ganoderma is a profound immune potentiator. It has been found to significantly improve the functioning of the immune system whether the immune system is deficient or excessive. In this sense, it is an immune "modulator" --- that is, it helps to modulate, or regulate, and fine tune the immune system. Our immune system is a virtually miraculous network of activities designed over millions of years to protect us from viruses, bacteria, parasites, molds, dust, pollen and malignant cells. It is the responsibility of the immune system to detect the intrusion, or invasion, of these entities and to mount a defense in order to eliminate them. A healthy immune system is capable of resisting most such intruders and a very hardy system may be able to resist invasions that many other people's systems cannot. If the immune system is weakened or malfunctioning, the invading microbes can easily establish a foothold in our body and disease sets in. Antibiotics can often be used to stop the invasion at this time, but chronic use of antibiotics further weakens the immune response. Furthermore, antibiotics are useless against viruses, pollens and most parasites. They are certainly useless against malignant (cancerous) cells generated in our own bodies. It is much better to resist the invasion from within with a fully fortified immune system and not become ill in the first place. This is where herbs like Reishi our now attracting the attention of scientists and consumers alike.

Many chemical constituents play a role in GL's immune modulating capacity. The polysaccharide components in particular seems to play an important role in attacking cancerous cells, but not healthy ones, while simultaneously strengthening the body's overall immune functions. The polysaccharides appear to help the body attack microbial invaders such as viruses, bacteria and yeast.

But Reishi does not just "stimulate" the immune system. It regulates it. And that is what makes Reishi so precious. If the immune system is excessive, as is the case with auto-immune diseases and allergies, Reishi can have significant positive influence. A group of chemicals known as the ganoderic acids help fight auto-immune diseases such as allergies. Ganoderic acids inhibit histamine release, improve oxygen utilization and improve liver functions. Ganoderic acids are also potent antioxidant free-radical scavengers.

Still another component, Beta-1, 3-glucan, helps regulate and stabilize blood sugar levels. Not only that, but these same components have been shown to have powerful anti-tumor properties.

Reishi is widely used in Asia to improve the cardiovascular system. It helps lower HDL (the "bad" cholesterol) and reduce excess fatty acids. It has been found to prevent and treat hardening of the arteries, angina and shortness of breath associated with coronary heart disease.

In 1977 it was discovered in Japan that Reishi had potent anti-cancer activity. It was first used to treat, and quite successfully, hairy-cell leukemia, which is caused by a retrovirus closely related to HIV, the virus that causes AIDS. It has been an approved drug for cancer in Japan since that time and has been used safely and effectively, often in conjunction with other drugs or radiation. It has been demonstrated that Reishi can help reduce the side-effects of many kinds of chemotherapy and radiation treatment and simultaneously contribute to the rebuilding of the immune system---an essential part of the recovery from cancer. Ganoderma stimulates the production of interferon and interleukins I and II, all being potent natural anti-cancer substances produced in our own bodies. Reishi may well prove to be the greatest prevention against cancer because it helps us to protect ourselves by our own power.

It has also been approved in Japan and China for the treatment of myasthenia gravis, a serious auto-immune disease. Besides that, it is commonly prescribed by MD.'s in Japan for chronic bronchitis, memory loss, insomnia, hyperlipidemia and a whole range of degenerative diseases of the elderly, including disorders associated with senility.

Reishi is a superb anti-stress herb. Throughout history it has been used to bring balance into the lives of people who needed help in this department, and that means most everyone. Deep in antiquity, it was routinely used by mountain hermits, monks, Taoist adepts and spiritual seekers throughout Asia because it was believed to help calm the mind, ease tension, strengthen the nerves, strengthen memory, sharpen concentration, improve focus, build will power and, as a result, help build wisdom. That is why it was called the "Mushroom of Spiritual Potency" by these seekers. The people of Asia have never lost their faith in Reishi. They believe more than ever in Reishi's power to improve the quality of life by improving the inner life of a human being. All the scientific validation only explains the physical nature of Reishi, but it is the profound ability of Reishi to improve one's life on every plane that makes it so miraculous. Reishi is indeed calming and centering. Everyone who takes Reishi notices the peacefulness that seems to accompany its use. Many people are able to stop using chemical drugs. And Reishi seems to be cumulative, gradually strengthening the nerves and actually changing how we perceive life.

Reishi is a substance that builds health on all levels. It is the rarest of jewels in Nature. Life itself is based on the ability to adapt to the stresses, the attacks, the challenges that come our way every day. Reishi seems to provide an incredible resource of the full range of energies we need to meet these challenges. Reishi is indeed "the great protector" protecting us on every level -- physically, immunologically, mentally, spiritually. It helps us adapt to the world and provides additional power for us to achieve a superior level of life. When we are so protected and so provided for, we can achieve things that otherwise would be impossible. That is why Reishi has been called the "herb of good fortune."

Thank You Note: The above information on the herbal properties of Reishi Mushroom, were taken from Ron Teeguarden's book Radiant Health, the Ancient Wisdom of the Chinese Tonic Herbs.

Organic Germanium

*Shelf fungus (Reishi Mushroom) has the highest content of organic germanium (2000-6000 ppm) and has a history of being an effective treatment for cancer. This was cited by Nobel Prize winner Alexander Solzhenitsyn in Cancer Ward. Garlic also has anti-tumor factor due to its content of organic germanium (754 ppm).

Organic germanium appears to play a role as an oxygen catalyst, an antioxidant, an electro-stimulant, and an immune enhancer.

Other researchers share the view that lack of oxygen to your cells, regardless of cause, leads to disease, unless appropriately checked. Among the proponents of this view are giants in the scientific community: Hans Selye, Albert Szent-Gyorgyi, Otto Warburg, and more recently, Stephen A. Levine and Parris M. Kidd. It may be that organic germanium can bring much needed oxygen to your cells.

A cell can, however, survive in the runaway, unhampered growth of cancer cells. This is called anaerobic metabolism as compared with aerobic metabolism. Aerobic cells live and grow in the presence of oxygen in an orderly, controlled pattern. Anaerobic cells grow in an uncontrolled pattern. Oxygen deprivation is considered to be its prime cause. The oxygen deficit leads to the anaerobic metabolism that sets the stage for the malignancy.

If cancer development is hampered in the presence of normal oxygen metabolism, organic germanium may be the supplement of choice as a cancer preventive.

Organic germanium may work as a catalyst, rather than a substitute, for oxygen. For reasons not yet understood, it has an oxygen sparing effect. It has been shown to lower the requirement for oxygen. The single most important substance for life - oxygen - may be the most powerful immune-stimulant of all.

Another role of organic germanium is that of detoxifier: It helps your body to expel pollutants. Because of its chelating effect, it is believed that organic germanium functions as an antioxidant as well as an oxidant.

Dr. Levine describes the role of oxygen as it relates to your electrical energy: "Like the electrical circuits in your home, your body is also electrical. Oxygen forms the positive terminal of your cellular battery. Energy from fresh natural foods provide current. Trace minerals, like selenium, zinc, iron, and manganese provide the wiring for the flow of electrical energy. Insulating material must coat and protect the energy transport machinery. For life, there must be a continuous flow of electricity, and adequate oxygen to draw the current."

Substances which help to normalize body functions indirectly are known as adaptogens. An adaptogen is classified as nontoxic and having a nonspecific effect, enhancing your ability to cope with any stress (physical, emotional, or chemical) as needed. Organic germanium has been reported to normalize acid/alkaline values, glucose curves, cholesterol levels, and blood pressure rates. Herbs like garlic, aloe, comfrey, chlorella and ginseng are adaptogens.

Studies confirming benefits of organic germanium

The Journal of Interferon Research 4 (1984):223-233. Organic germanium restores the normal function of T-cells, B-lymphocytes, antibody-dependent cell toxicity, natural killer cell activity, and the numbers of antibody-forming cells. Studies indicate that this compound has unique physiological activities without any significant toxic effects. Organic germanium has the ability to modulate alterations in the immune response.

Tokyo Electric Hospital of Opthalmology, Dr Akira Ishikawa. Eye manifestations are closely related with systemic diseases. Decrease in in retinal blood pressure was observed with administration of organic germanium. (This was the first report of the use of organic germanium in the field of opthalmology.) It is also effective in the treatment and prevention of essential hypertension and diabetes by effecting a normalization of the body state.

Journal of Pharmacological Dynamics 6 (1983):814-820. Organic germanium enhances morphine analgesia in both oral administration and injection. It appears to act by increasing the activity of morphine at the receptor sites, and by releasing self-made endorphins (the morphine-like substances manufactured by humans).

Cancer and Chemotherapy 6, in Japanese (1968):79-83. Organic germanium demonstrates antitumor activity.

Gan to Kagaku Ryoho 12, December 1985:2345-51. A remarkable prolongation of life span is observed after oral administration of organic germanium.

Anticancer Research 6, March-April 1986:177-82. Organic germanium administered to test animals with tumors results in the inhibition of tumor growth.

Gan to Kagaku Ryoho 12, November 1985:2122-8. Organic germanium-treated test animals show an inhibitory effect against certain tumors in such a way that suggest that the effect is the result of macrophage activity. (Macrophages are part of the immune system. They attack the enemy.)

Anticancer Research 5, Sept.-Oct. 1985:479-83. Test animals were inoculated with carcinoma or leukemia cells, and then treated orally with organic germanium. The study demonstrates that the effect of organic germanium work through the body's mechanisms (including macrophages and/or T-cells) rather than attacking the cancer itself.

Gan to Kagaku Ryoho 13, Aug. 1986:2588-93. This study suggests that organic germanium is useful for antitumor combination immunochemotherapy. The results are an inhibition of tumor growth, enhanced anti-metastatic effect, prolonged survival time, and recovery of lost body weight caused by chemotherapy.

Tohoku Journal of Experimental Medicine 146, May 1985:97-104. The antitumor action of organic germanium appears to be related to its interferon-inducing activity.

Reference: Germanium, A New Approach to Immunity, by Betty Kamen, 1987.

"There is nothing which heaven does not cover, yet nothing that earth does not sustain." -- Chuang Tzu

There needs to be a balance and integration between the heavenly *yang* therapies such as Qi-healing, Qigong and acupuncture with the earthly *yin* aspect such as diet and tonic superior herbs which together create harmony, healing wholeness of yin and yang and spiritual oneness with the universe to truely envision what Taoist master Chuang Tzu said, "There is nothing which heaven does not cover, yet nothing that earth does not sustain."

Tonic herbs are herbs which promote a long, healthy, vibrant, happy life without any unwanted side effects even when taken over a long period of time. The tonic or Superior Herbs, essentially, are empowering and healthful "super-foods" which benefit our well-being in ways that more common foods cannot. And they have a protective, balancing, vitalizing quality beyond that of any other herbs. They are generally consumed as a herbal supplement to a well-balanced healthy diet for the purpose of optimizing our nutritional needs

Applying the principle of the Three Treasures is the highest form of great herbalism. (Three Treasures) In the Orient it is called "the Superior Herbalism." Six tonic or superior herbs revered by the great sages as the quintessential substances to cultivate the Three Treasures (Qi, Shen, and Jing) are Reishi mushrooms, Ginseng, Schizandra fruit (Wu Wei Zi), Asparagus Root (Tian Men Dong), Gynostemma Pentaphyllum (Jiao Gu Lan), and Rhodiola (Hong Jing Tian). Shen Nong Ben Cao (Divine Farmer's Materia Medica) and Huang Di Neijing (Yellow Emperor's Classic of Medicine) described them as superior or immortal foods as opposed to the medicinal and radical herbs.

Guo Lin Qigong with Tonic Herbs

A form of Qigong that builds the Three Treasures and complements the six tonic herbs or superior herbs is called Guo Lin New Qigong.

Guo Lin qigong is a Kidney protection Qigong that helps to heal cancer, kidney diseases, diabetes, lung diseases, infertility, hydronephrosis, and cardiovascular diseases.

What is Guo Lin Qigong?

Also known as "Walking Qigong", was invented by Guo Lin (1909-1984).

Guo Lin was diagnosed with cancer in the 1940s and underwent extensive surgery. Using the traditional Qi Gong her grandfather had taught her and her knowledge of TCM, she developed a new form to aid in her recovery now known as Guo Lin Qi Gong. After a full recovery she began to teach to the public.

Following the success enjoyed by many other patients, in 1977 she approached the National Health Department to advocate a new approach to cancer combining the strengths of western medicine, traditional Chinese medicine and Guo Lin Qi Gong.

In 1982, with government support, she built a new hospital to carry her work further which has assisted thousands of cancer patients. Guo Lin died in 1984 of a sudden stroke.

The use of chi gong for cancer treatment in China originated with Ms. Guo Lin, a Chinese traditional painter, mentioned above. In 1949, she was afflicted with uterine cancer and had it removed by surgery in Shanghai. The cancer recurred in 1960. This time it had metastasized to the bladder, and she had another operation in Beijing to remove part of the bladder that was cancerous. When she had another relapse, the doctors gave her six months to live. However, she did not give up hope, and in her struggle against cancer, she remembered that her grandfather, a Taoist priest, had taught her as a child to practice chi gong. She determinedly began to research and practice chi gong, hoping to recover her health in this way. After initial practice with no effect, she turned to the ancient chi gong texts willed to her by her grandfather and created her own exercise schedule. She practiced diligently for two hours every day, and in half a year her cancer subsided. She was strongly convinced of chi gong's ability to cure diseases, and in 1970 started giving lessons in what she called New Chi Gong Therapy. According to Cyrus Lee, Master Guo's therapy is not based on the external energy (wei chi) of others, but upon the inner energy (nei chi) of the patient (for these distinctions, review chapter 1, "Special Section on Chi"). Her therapy combines "active and passive exercises in three stages: relaxation (sung jing), concentration (yi lian), and breathing (tiao hsi)."[2]

By 1977 Master Guo had achieved spectacular results and proclaimed publicly that chi gong can cure cancer. Cancer victims from all over immediately streamed into Beijing to take part in the chi gong cancer therapy class she had organized. Each day three hundred to four hundred people studied chi gong techniques for cancer treatment with her. Until her death in 1984 she worked tirelessly, curing hundreds of cancer patients, while easing the pain and prolonging the lives of thousands more. Mrs. Wong Chung-siu, a student of Guo Lin's currently living in Fremont, California, told Paul Dong that Guo Lin's pinnacle of success came in 1982. Aided by nine assistants she had trained, Guo Lin held nine cancer classes of seventy students each, meeting three times a day. With her nine assistants to help her, she was able over the next two years to travel all over China to twenty provincial capitals to teach and lecture at the request of many local health care and medical departments, and she became a national celebrity before her death in 1984 (twenty years after her life had been given up by Western medicine).

Because Guo Lin had demonstrated that her chi gong techniques were able to cure cancer, people trained in other styles of chi gong were eager to see if they could achieve the same results. Among these other styles, quiet gong and movement gong also demonstrated the same ability to achieve cures or alleviation of cancer. Paul Dong judges from the Chinese literature that movement gong is more effective in curing cancer. The technique used by Guo Lin combines both movement chi gong and meditation chi gong (movement first and quiet gong afterward).

Foot Notes:

1. Ke Yan, "Cancer Does Not Mean Death," Beijing Literature, July 1982, 43.

2. Cyrus Lee, "Qi Gong (Breath Exercise) and Its Major Models," Chinese Cukure 24 (September1984): 71-79. The description was Quoted by Prof. Lee from Guo Lin's book Hsin Qigong Liao Fa (Hofei: Science and Technology Press, 1980), 4.

Read Therapeutic Breathing, page 53; How Guo Lin Qigong works, pages 55-56; Testimonials, page 57; Get Well Verse for Cancer patients, page 112; and Introduction to Guo Lin Qigong, page 120.

Dr Budwig Diet for Cancer and Degenerative Diseases

"The essential fatty acids are at the core of the answer to the cancer problem." Dr. Robert Willner, MD, PhD., The Cancer Solution

INTRODUCTORY NOTE by Ricardo B Serrano, R.Ac.: For best healing results of chronic diseases such as cancer, heart disease, stroke, arthritis, and other diseases, the simple Diet of Dr. Johanna Budwig - cottage cheese and Flaxseed oil combined with flax seeds - builds the Ka pranic body, Qi life-force, and Jing (essence), and can be integrated with meditation, Qigong, and other Oriental medical treatments together with *Virgin Coconut Oil*.

Johanna Budwig (30 September 1908; 19 May 2003) was a German chemist, pharmacologist and physicist. She developed and promoted (from 1952) the Budwig protocol/Budwig diet, which centres around the regular consumption of foods rich in linolenic and linoleic acids.

The two unsaturated fatty acids have 3 high-energy double bonds (pi-electrons). These fatty acids affect the membranes of cells and are believed to affect oxygen transport and assimilation. Budwig's concept was that the omega-3 and omega-6 fatty acids act to repair damaged cell walls and affect chemical communication of cancer cells to the point where they normalize.

Flaxseed oil (cold-pressed, unprocessed) and low fat cottage cheese are the mainstay of Budwig's cancer diet (also used for heart disease) (cottage cheese has actually become to be used as a more readily-available substitute for the quark cheese which Johanna Budwig had used in her original work).

In addition to the above components, the Budwig diet advocates the consumption of organic vegetable juices (most prominently carrot juice) and polyphenols such as resveratrol (found in red wine). The diet bans consumption of animal and hydrogenated fats, foods high in preservatives, meats, and especially sugar. She advocated the consumption of whole foods which contain antioxidants in their natural form.

Budwig claimed this diet would cure or prevent many forms of cancers, particularly breast and prostate cancer, and a long list of other degenerative disease including cardiovascular diseases and skin diseases.

"Numerous, independent clinical studies published in major medical journals world-wide confirm Dr. Budwig's findings

... Over 40 years ago Dr Budwig presented clear and convincing evidence, which has been confirmed by hundreds of other related scientific research papers since, that the essential fatty acids were at the core of the answer to the cancer problem ... You will come to your own conclusions as to why this simple effective prevention and therapy has not only been ignored it has been suppressed!" - Dr Robert Willner, M.D., Ph.D. (The Cancer Solution)

According to the Budwig Diet by Dr. Robert Willner, "Six time nobel award nominated doctor says this essential nutrient combination actually prevents and cures cancer!

A top European cancer research scientist, Dr Johanna Budwig, has discovered a totally natural formula that not only protects against the development of cancer but people all over the world who have been diagnosed with incurable cancer and sent home to die have actually been cured and now lead normal healthy lives.

After three decades of research Dr. Budwig, six-time nominee for the Nobel Award, found that the blood of seriously ill cancer patients was always, without exception, deficient in certain important essential ingredients which included substances called phosphatides and lipoproteins. (The blood of a healthy person always contains sufficient quantities of these essential ingredients. However, without these natural ingredients cancer cells grow wild and out of control.)

Blood analysis showed a strange greenish-yellow substance in place of the healthy red oxygen carrying hemoglobin that belongs there. This explained why cancer patients weaken and become anemic This startling discovery led Dr. Budwig to test her theory.

She found that when these natural ingredients where replaced over approximately a three month period, tumors gradually receded. The strange greenish elements in the blood were replaced with healthy red blood cells as the phosphatides and lipoproteins almost miraculously reappeared. Weakness and anemia disappeared and life energy was restored. Symptoms of cancer, liver dysfunction and diabetes were completely alleviated.

Dr. Budwig then discovered an all-natural way for people to replace those essential ingredients their bodies so desperately needed in their daily diet. By simply eating a combination of just two natural and delicious foods not only can cancer be prevented but in case after case it was actually cured. (These two natural foods, organic flax seed oil & cottage cheese) must be eaten together to be effective since one triggers the properties of the other to be released.)

After more than 10 years of solid clinical application, Dr. Budwig's natural formula has proven successful where many orthodox remedies have failed. Dr. Budwig's formula has been used therapeutically in Europe for prevention of: Cancer! Arteriosclerosis, Strokes, Cardiac Infarction, Heartbeat (irregular), Liver (fatty degeneration), Lungs (reduces bronchial spasms), Intestines (regulates activity), Stomach Ulcers (normalizes gastric juices), Prostate (hypertopic), Arthritis (exerts a favorable influence), Eczema (assists all skin diseases), Old age (improves many common afflictions), Brain (strengthens activity), Immune Deficiency Syndromes (multiple sclerosis, auto-immune illnesses).

Thousands have flocked to hear Dr. Budwig lecture all over Europe. The many people Dr. Budwig's formula has helped testify to the benefits of her remarkable discovery. Following are a few examples: In one of my interviews with Dr. Budwig I was introduced to Siegfried Ernst, M.D.. He is a rare and dedicated man who counts among his personal friends the current Pope as well as many other dignitaries.

Seventeen years ago Dr. Ernst had developed cancer for which he had major surgery requiring removal of his stomach. Two years later he had a recurrence of the cancer and was offered chemotherapy as the only available remedy. There was little hope for survival as virtually all individuals with recurrence of this type of cancer rarely last a year.

Dr. Ernst knew that chemotherapy was not only ineffective for his type of cancer but completely destructive of the quality of life, so he refused.

He turned to Dr. Budwig and her formula for help. He religiously followed Dr. Budwig's formula and fifteen years later has not had any recurrence of cancer. As a matter of fact he seemed to me to be in perfect health and is tireless for a man in his late seventies.

Maria W. tells her story in her own words: "I was told by the most expert of doctors that I would have to be operated on to cut out the cancerous tumor that was causing a swelling under my eye. They explained that the size of the tumor was much greater inside and that there was very serious bone involvement. The malignancy was too far advanced to respond to radiation treatment. The doctors planned to remove considerable facial tissue and bone. I was afraid for my life, but being a young woman, couldn't bear the thought of such disfigurement.

When I heard about Dr. Budwig's natural formula, I was skeptical but desperate for help. After four months on this regimen, the swelling under my left eye completely disappeared. The doctors at the University hospital gave me many exhausting tests. One told me, 'If I didn't have your previous x-rays and medical history in front of me, I wouldn't believe that you ever had cancer. There is hardly any indication of a tumor remaining.' I never thought using Dr, Budwig's formula would be so successful. My whole family and I are very grateful."

An examination of Sandy A. revealed arachnoidal bleeding due to an inoperable brain tumor. The doctors informed Sandy that he was beyond medical help. At his expressed wish, Sandy was discharged from the hospital and sent home to die in peace.

A friend brought Dr. Budwig's formula to Sandy's attention. Sandy writes. "Since I went on the Budwig regimen, the paralysis is of my eyes, arms, and legs has receded daily. After only a short period of time, I was able to urinate normally. My health improved so rapidly that I was soon able to return to my work part-time. Shortly after that, I was again examined at the Research Center and my reflexes were completely normal. The Budwig diet saved my life! Ten years later, I was given a thorough examination at the Center as a follow-up. My incredible recovery has been written up In many medical journals and I have become what they call a 'text-book case,' and all because of Dr. Johanna Budwig's simple diet."

Seven years ago Timmy G. was diagnosed as having Hodgkins disease. The child was operated on and underwent 24 radiation treatments, plus additional experimental therapies that the experts hoped would be of some small help. When Timmy failed to respond favorably to these heroic measures, he was discharged as incurable, and given six months to live and sent home to die.

The desperate parents contacted specialists all over the world. A famous newspaper took up Timmy's cause and ran editorials pleading for someone to come forth who could offer hope for the life of a child. All the specialists who replied confirmed the cruel prognosis: There was no hope or help for Timmy. At this dark hour the miracle the family had prayed for happened! Timmy's mother told her story to the press:

"A friend sent me a printed piece about one of Dr. Budwig's speeches. This material gave us hope and I contacted Dr. Budwig.

In just five days, (on the Budwig regimen) Timmy's breathing became normal for the first time in almost two years. From this day on, Timmy began to feel good again. He went back to school, started swimming and by winter he was doing craft work. Everyone who knows him says how well he looks." At age 18 Timmy is showing great promise in his university work. He knows he owes his life to Dr. Budwig and thanks her daily in his prayers.

One of the two foods in on Budwig's formula, cottage cheese, is available in nearly every grocery store in America. The other, pure organic linseed oil, however comes primarily from Europe and can only be found in certain health food stores throughout the United States.

By simply mixing these two delicious foods together and eating them you will be providing yourself and your family with the optimal preventive nutritional protection against cancer and other disease."

Quotations from other holistic Doctors:

"What she (Dr. Johanna Budwig) has demonstrated to my initial disbelief but lately, to my complete satisfaction in my practice is: CANCER IS EASILY CURABLE, the treatment is dietary/lifestyle, the response is immediate; the cancer cell is weak and vulnerable; the precise biochemical breakdown point was identified by her in 1951 and is specifically correctable, in vitro (test-tube) as well as in vivo (real)... " Dr. Dan C. Roehm M.D. FACP (Oncologist and former cardiologist) in 1990 http://www.oxytherapy.com/mail-archive/oct96/165.html

"Cancer patients suffer from a faulty metabolism caused by a malfunction in the lipid defense system. By repairing the lipid defense system the cancer cannot survive. Of course common chemo and radiation causes further harm to the lipid defense system - the very system that protects you from cancer! The folks who will READILY ADMIT that they don't understand the cancer mechanism will tell you with their next breath that cancer can be killed with poisons. So can you. Would you trust your car to a so-called mechanic who didn't understand what makes a car work properly? If not, why would you let someone who doesn't understand cancer "fix" your body? The average cancer docs don't know -- they admit it. That doesn't make them bad people, it just makes them unqualified to treat your condition if you have cancer. Don't let unqualified people poison you just because they don't know what else to do". - William Kelley Eidem, author "The Doctor Who Cures Cancer (Dr Revici)

"I have the answer to cancer, but American doctors won't listen. They come here and observe my methods and are impressed. Then they want to make a special deal so they can take it home and make a lot of money. I won't do it, so I'm blackballed in every country." - Dr Budwig.

"Nobody seemed to notice that a crime has been committed: It was the case of the missing nutrient. The nutrient was essential; it was a nutrient we human beings needed in order to stay healthy. It started to disappear from our diet about 75 years ago and now is almost gone. Only about 20% of the amount needed for human health and well-being remains. The nutrient is a fatty acid so important and so little understood that I call it "the nutritional missing link" ... Food grade linseed oil & fish oil are the best sources of this special fat - Omega 3 essential fatty acid - which modern food destroys." - Donaldo. Rudin, M.D. (The Omega 3 Phenomenon)

In a 1994 study of 121 women with breast cancer, those in more advanced stages whose breast cancer had spread to their lymph nodes showed the lowest levels of omega-3 fatty acids in the breast tissue. After 31 months, the 20 women who had developed metastases had significantly lower levels of these EFAs (Essential fatty acids) than those who didn't. Another study out of Boston University using the same type of tissue profiles that were used in the breast cancer study demonstrated that patients with coronary artery disease likewise had, low levels of EFAs.

"The association between fats - meaning saturated, refined w6s (Omega 6), rancid fats, processed oils, and altered fats - and cancer, (but excluding w3s and fresh, natural, unrefined oils) has long been documented. (They) interfere with oxygen use in our cells. Heat, hydrogenation, light, and oxygen produce chemically altered fat products that are toxic to our cells ... These fats kill people. Healing fats in cancer include ... w3s (Omega 3s), enhance oxygen use in cells, decrease tumour formation, slow tumour growth, decrease tumour formation, decrease the spread of cancer cells (metastasis), and extend the patient's survival time. Unsaturated fatty acids in fresh, unheated oils are anti-mutagenic ... W9, w6, w3 are all effective. Saturated fatty acids to not have this protective ability. Heating these oils above 150C makes them lose their protective power, and they become mutation-causing. ALL mass market oils except virgin olive oil have undergone heating during deodorization ... When we use virgin olive oil or other unrefined oils for sauteeing, frying ... we overheat them, destroying their protective, anti-mutagenic properties. ALL hydrogenated and partially hydrogenated products have also been overheated.." - Udo Erasmus (Fats That Heal, Fats That Kill).

"Our immune system, which is vital for destroying cancer cells, requires EFAs, vitamins C, B6, and A, and zinc to function, and requires an exceptionally rich nutrient supply of ALL essential nutrients for its high level of complex cellular activities. Deficiencies of EFAs and toxic, man-made synthetic drugs that interfere with essential fatty acid functions can create the conditions of fatty degeneration collectively known as cancer." - Erasmus

Dr Rudin believes the Omega 3 story parallels the story of Beriberi & Pellagra. It took them 200 years to accept pellagra was a nutrient deficiency.

"Compared to 100 years ago, Omega 3 is down 80%, B vitamins are estimated to be down to about 50% of the daily requirement. Vitamin B6 consumption may be low as it is removed in grain milling and not replaced. Vitamins B1, B2, B3 and E have also been lost in food processing. Minerals are depleted in a similar way. Fibre is down 75-80%. Antinutrients have increased substantially---saturated fat, 100%; cholestrol, 50%; refined sugar nearly 1000%; salt up to 500%; and funny fat isomers nearly 1,000%." - Dr Rudin.

"Dr. Budwig's diet is the best diet for the prevention and cure of cancer and chronic diseases because it builds the Ka pranic body, Qi life-force and Jing. Flaxseed oil and fish oil are both Yin and Jing tonics that along with Chinese tonic herbs help to strengthen the kidneys, which store and consolidate the Jing. In Chinese medicine, Jing is our essence, it's the quality of our genetic heritage from our parents. As we age, we slowly use up our Jing and we die when our Jing is extinguished." - Ricardo B Serrano, R.Ac.

Quotations from Lothar Hirneise' Chemotherapy Heals Cancer and the World is Flat:

"A tumour is an incredibly ingenious solution on the part of the body."

"Every successful cancer treatment contains three ingredients: thorough detoxification, a change of diet and mental or spiritual work."

"Of course chemotherapy is no fun, but a radical change in your diet and lifestyle is more difficult. That's why so few people survive cancer."

"Cancer cannot exist without stress. One hundred percent impossible!"

"For me the oil-protein diet always serves as the basis of a cancer therapy and please understand that I am not just simply writing this, but that I have carefully chosen my words, as I have become familiar with more than 100 different alternative cancer therapies in recent years, and I have investigated many of them. When Dr. Johanna Budwig died the cancer scene lost one of the last great scientists of the last century, and it behoves each of us to carry her legacy to future generations, so that they as well can profit from the oil-protein diet."

CONCLUDING NOTE by Ricardo B Serrano, R.Ac.: The Budwig Diet that is rich in phosphatides and lipoproteins which are missing in today's standard diet has been used for over 60 years with astonishing curative healing effects to most chronic diseases including cancer. Food is the best medicine, according to Oriental medicine. The Budwig diet (The Cancer Solution) and Ketogenic Diet with Virgin Coconut Oil consumption integrated with lifestyle dietary change, Chinese tonic herbs, meditation, emotional stress healing, Qi-healing, acupressure, acupuncture, exercise, and Qigong therapy have proven to greatly heal clients with cancer and other chronic health problems for over half a century and will be therapeutically used in the coming years as safe viable alternative holistic approach. With these powerful knowledge at your disposal now, disregard your unnecessary fear because you have the keys to healing.

Book References: Cancer: The Problem and the Solution by Dr. Johanna Budwig and Lothar Hirneise, 2008. The Cancer Solution by Dr. Robert E. Willner, MD, PhD., 1993.

Co-factors in Fat Metabolism

In the metabolism of fats, several minerals and vitamins are known to be involved. The involvements of many others is not yet certain. This field of study, important as it is, is just in its infancy.

In order to break down saturated fatty acids into 2-carbon fragments (beta-oxidation), several co-factors are required, because many different enzyme steps are involved. Vitamins B2, B3, pantothenic acid, sulphur, and potassium are all required in different steps of the break-down process of these saturated fatty acids.

To synthesize fatty acids out of 2-carbon fragments, vitamins B2, B3, and biotin are necessary co-factors. In burning the 2-carbon fragments into carbon dioxide and water, vitamins B2, B3, and iron act as co-factors. Inserting cis- double bonds into saturated fatty acid molecules also requires vitamins B2 and B3, and iron as co-factors.

To change linoleic acid (18:2w6) into prostaglandins E1, several enzymes are involved, and each enzyme has its own co-factor requirement. The first requires zinc, and is blocked by excess fats, cholesterol, saturated fatty acids, processed vegetable oils, and alcohol. The second step requires vitamin B6, The third step requires zinc, vitamin B3, and vitamin C. If any of these co-factors are missing, some step in the manufacture of prostaglandin E1 is blocked. If any of the co-factors are in short supply, the production of prostaglandin E1 is slowed down. Lack or low level of prostaglandin E1 is a factor in many physical and several mental ailments and its symptoms are similar to those of essential fatty acid deficiency and degenerative diseases.

For transport in the body, cholesterol needs to be hooked (esterified) to a fatty acid, preferably an essential fatty acid. Esterification requires vitamin B6. To change cholesterol into bile acids, vitamin C is required. Vitamin B3 is involved in regulating blood cholesterol level, though the exact role B3 plays in regulation is not yet known.

From these short, partial list of examples, we can see that many essential nutritional factors are required for fat metabolism. These have to be supplied through the diet in sufficient, or even better, in optimal quantities. If we don't get them, the metabolism of fats and oils cannot take place the way it should, and when that happens we lose health and vigour.

Deranged fat metabolism lies at the root of most degenerative diseases. This derangement may be caused by too much of the wrong kinds of fats in our diet, too much total fat, or deficiency of the right kinds of fats. It may also be the deficiency of any of the necessary co-factors that deranges fat metabolism. That's why all of the nutritional factors have to be in place, working together.

One example will illustrate this point. Cancer is the enigma of our time, eluding every attempt at pin-pointing its exact cause, which is often assumed to be a single cause. It clearly is a form of fatty degeneration, something gone haywire with the way the cells handle fats and energy production.

There may be changes in the fat composition of cell membranes, there may be fat droplets within the cells, or there may be fats surrounding the tumor. In separate animal experiments, it has been shown that cancer can be induced by an imbalance in any one of many factors. Deficiency of essential fatty acids, too much saturated fatty acids, too many calories, deficiency of zinc, iron, oxygen, vitamin A, vitamin C, vitamin B1, B2, B6, pantothenic acid, vitamin E, sulphur, protein deficiency (especially the amino acid methionine) and perhaps choline deficiency can lead to cancer. The list may not be complete. Similarly, it has been shown that a diet rich in these factors protects animals from radiation-induced and chemically-induced cancers.

Co-factor Deficiencies

Surveys of human nutritional states have uncovered that the most common deficiencies among humans are vitamins C, E, and A, and the minerals iron, zinc, calcium, and magnesium. Essential fatty acid deficiency and deficiencies of the B vitamins are widespread. Iodine and manganese deficiencies are also common. Nutritional surveys in America showed that between 60 and 80% of the population is deficient in one or more essential nutrients. Over 75% of the people die from degenerative diseases.

It does not take much imagination to put these pieces of information together. The vitamin and mineral co-factors of fat metabolism deserve more attention. Our diet needs to be complete, needs to contain all of the essential elements of nutrition working together to maintain health, and a vigorous, long life.

Cancer is fatty degeneration.

Cancer is fatty degeneration. Microscopic studies have revealed that the common feature of all types of cancer cells is the presence of fatty materials within the cell plasma and the nucleus. These findings have been confirmed by electron microscopic examination in France. The fats do not appear to take part in cell functions. Healthy cells are free of them.

Hard tumors have a hard, rubbery, sulphur-containing proteinaceous core, surrounded by oils which cannot form associations with the proteins. These two essential elements which belong together are separate because the oils are denatured, altered, unable to fulfill their biological functions.

Dr. Budwig considers cancer to be not cell growth out of control, but retarded. Her basis for saying so is that in rapidly growing tissues, one always finds high concentration of essential fatty acids and high oxygen consumption, whereas in tumors, essential fatty acid concentration and oxygen consumption are always depressed. The pile-up of tumor material is the result of debris which the cell cannot take away because it lacks the energy necessary to do so. This energy is supplied by essential fatty acids and oxygen (along with the other essential nutrients.

Cancer represents the most extreme form of nutritional collapse. The metabolic rate is decreased. Oxygen uptake is inhibited. Cell division often remains incomplete. The polarity of the cells is disrupted and all the cell's functions are crippled. The membranes are defective. The red blood cells fall apart. The cell is in a severe state of disorganization.

Long chain saturated fatty acids interfere with oxygen use in the cell, as do altered fatty acids and fat products created by processing seed and marine animal oils. Heat, hydrogenation, light, and oxygen all produce chemically altered fat products which are toxic to the cell. Products altered by processing include margarines, shortening, partially hydrogenated oils, deep friend oils, refined, deodorized oils, oils exposed to light in transparent bottles on store shelves, oils fried in the home, and oils gone rancid from exposure to oxygen after opening the bottle.

Fatty acids which enhance oxygen use in the cells and which help to dissolve tumors are the essential fatty acids found in the fresh seeds of flax, pumpkin, soy bean, and walnut, or their fresh oils from these seeds. These fatty acids are also found in the fish oils of the fatty fish, while those fish are fresh.

Deficiency of the co-factors required to protect the highly unsaturated fatty acids from damage, or required to metabolize the fatty acids from damage, or required to metabolize the fatty acids and sugars also interferes with oxygen use in the cells. Co-factors include several B-complex vitamins required for the production, by oxidation of energy within the cell, the vitamin E and A, which protect the integrity of the highly unsaturated fatty acids and the cell membranes, and vitamins C, B3 and B6, the minerals zinc, selenium, and iron, and sulphur-containing amino acids, which facilitate the production of prostaglandins. Deficiency of any one of these can disrupt metabolism enough to cause the fatty degeneration called cancer. The immune system, vital for destroying cancer cells, require essential fatty acids, vitamin C, B6, and zinc to function.

Finally, many man-made synthetic drugs, which interfere with the functions of the essential fatty acids, and deficiencies of the fatty acids themselves, can also create the conditions of fatty degeneration collectively known as cancer.

Other conditions of fatty degeneration diseases are obesity, diabetes, rheumatism, acne, multiple sclerosis, cystic fibrosis, fatty degeneration conditions of the liver (cirrhosis), the kidneys, the heart and other internal organs, glandular atrophy, arthritis, asthma, food allergies, premenstrual syndrome and breast pain, many liver and gall problems, calcium metabolism, cellulite, various problems of sense organs, brown spots on the skin called aging spots or cemetery flowers, deposition of fatty material under the eyes and on the white of the eye ball

One Cause? Can it be possible that so many different conditions have one underlying cause? The common underlying factor is the excess saturated fats and sugars in our diets, excess altered fats and fat-like substances, and an inadequate supply of essential fatty acids in their natural state.

The reason for this common underlying problem rests in the consumption of refined foods in which the essential fatty acids have been systematically destroyed, removed, or altered during processing practices. The essential fatty acids would spoil (and do spoil) on the shelf if left in the food. The blame for the consumption of deficient foods, although these are offered to us by producers, processors, and manufacturers, lies with us, the consumers. We buy and eat these foods. We make the choices, and we change the choices when they no longer work for us, and when we know better. There are, after all, people living in this society, who do not acquire, and who do not live in fear of acquiring, any of the afflictions of fatty degeneration. Their immunity lies in their food choices and lifestyle. There are, furthermore, people who, having become ill with one of the degenerative diseases, have had the will to stop, to search, to learn, to change, and to heal themselves. This too, is possible.

Differences, Too

On the other hand, the underlying causes for the diseases of fatty degeneration are not all the same. Besides the common denominator of the faulty consumption and metabolism of fats, there are also differences. Other nutritional deficiencies come into play. Deficiency of zinc will cause degeneration in a way that is different than deficiency of vitamin C, but both will cause disease. That is why, beyond the fatty part of the degeneration, the different members of the degenerative family also show differences in their symptoms and treatment.

Individual differences also determine whether a person gets one kind of fatty degeneration or another. Every person has some stronger and some weaker organs. The weaker organs are the first to be affected by deficiency. People are also different in their requirements of different nutrients,

Finally, other factors, such as different drugs that people take, the kind and amounts of alcohol, cigarettes, fresh air, and sunshine they consume, how much exercise they get, how much joy they have, what their mental program is, all determine how well a person's body will cope with living in the world, with stress and with challenge.

Source: Fats and Oils by Udo Erasmus, 1986.

Glutathione in Health and Disease

It is believed that glutathione has a potential role to play in the treatment and prevention of hundreds of diseases. It may in the future be considered as important to health as a well-documented diet, exercise and good lifestyle. Clinical tests show that raised glutathione levels may address some of the major health issues of our time - heart disease, stroke, diabetes, high cholesterol, asthma, cigarette smoking, hepatitis, cancer, Parkinson's, Alzheimer's, AIDS, and more. Glutathione provides the body with tools to fight off these threats naturally.

Putting it all together

- Medical science is still ascertaining all the critical roles played by glutathione in disease resistance and general good health. Clinical evidence links low glutathione levels to the most common illnesses of our times as well as newly emerging diseases.
- As an essential AID to health, glutathione works as a master Antioxidant in our body, optimizes the Immune system and Detoxifies a long list of pollutants and carcinogens. However, the body's glutathione levels are not raised by eating glutathione, since it is poorly absorbed through the digestive system. It must be manufactured within the cells of the body. Therefore, the best way to raise glutathione is by providing the building blocks used by the cells to make it themselves.

- Pharmaceutical medicine has created drugs *NAC* (n-acetyl-cysteine) that do this very effectively, and they have their uses in clinical situations. But they also have side effects and repeated use is clearly inadvisable. Recently, scientists have developed a natural way to raise glutathione levels by safe, reliable dietary means. The emergence of bioactive whey proteins is an exciting step forward in nutritional supplementation.

Bioactive Whey Protein

Bioactive whey proteins contain high levels of non-denatured protein and this assures their glutathione-promoting activity. Much of our knowledge of the glutathione sustaining effect of dietary whey proteins is the result of research initiated at Montreal's McGill University in Canada during the early 1980's. Dr. Gustavo Bounous was studying protein supplementation in general when he discovered the bioactive potential of whey protein in particular. He investigated its effect on the immune system and published his ground-breaking results. They encouraged other scientific teams to study the effects of glutathione-enhancement in tests on a wide variety of diseases. Dr. Bounous and his team went on to develop *Immunocal* - a whey protein made under pharmacological conditions to maximize the protein's bioactivity.

Undenatured whey protein is a natural extract of milk - a safe, dependable and effective way to sustain elevated glutathione levels.

What's the connection between glutathione and cancer?

Glutathione helps us fight cancer in at least three ways: Firstly and most importantly, it can prevent cancers from developing in the first place. Secondly, glutathione tends to combat cancers already established in the body. Lastly, it can alleviate many of the consequences of cancer, including severe weight loss, and the side effects of chemotherapy and radiation.

Coconut In Traditional Medicine

People from many diverse cultures, languages, religions, and races scattered around the globe have revered the coconut as a valuable source of both food and medicine. Wherever the coconut palm grows the people have learned of its importance as a effective medicine. For thousands of years coconut products have held a respected and valuable place in local folk medicine.

In traditional medicine around the world coconut is used to treat a wide variety of health problems including the following: abscesses, asthma, baldness, bronchitis, bruises, burns, colds, constipation, cough, dropsy, dysentery, earache, fever, flu, gingivitis, gonorrhea, irregular or painful menstruation, jaundice, kidney stones, lice, malnutrition, nausea, rash, scabies, scurvy, skin infections, sore throat, swelling, syphilis, toothache, tuberculosis, tumors, typhoid, ulcers, upset stomach, weakness, and wounds.

Coconut Oil

While coconut possesses many health benefits due to its fiber and nutritional content, it's the oil that makes it a truly remarkable food and medicine.

Once mistakenly believed to be unhealthy because of its high saturated fat content, it is now known that the fat in coconut oil is a unique and different from most all other fats and possesses many health giving properties. It is now gaining long overdue recognition as a nutritious health food.

Coconut oil has been described as "the healthiest oil on earth." That's quite a remarkable statement. What makes coconut oil so good? What makes it different from all other oils, especially other saturated fats?

The difference is in the fat molecule. All fats and oils are composed of molecules called fatty acids. There are two methods of classifying fatty acids. The first you are probably familiar with, is based on saturation. You have saturated fats, monounsaturated fats, and polyunsaturated fats. Another system of classification is based on molecular size or length of the carbon chain within each fatty acid. Fatty acids consist of long chains of carbon atoms with hydrogen atoms attached. In this system you have short-chain fatty acids (SCFA), medium-chain fatty acids (MCFA), and long-chain fatty acids (LCFA). Coconut oil is composed predominately of medium-chain fatty acids (MCFA), also known as medium-chain triglycerides (MCT).

The vast majority of fats and oils in our diets, whether they are saturated or unsaturated or come from animals or plants, are composed of long-chain fatty acids (LCFA). Some 98 to 100% of all the fatty acids you consume are LCFA.

The size of the fatty acid is extremely important. Why? Because our bodies respond to and metabolize each fatty acid differently depending on its size. So the physiological effects of MCFA in coconut oil are distinctly different from those of LCFA more commonly found in our foods. The saturated fatty acids in coconut oil are predominately medium-chain fatty acids. Both the saturated and unsaturated fat found in meat, milk, eggs, and plants (including most all vegetable oils) are composed of LCFA. MCFA are very different from LCFA. They do not have a negative effect on cholesterol and help to protect against heart disease. MCFA help to lower the risk of both atherosclerosis and heart disease. It is primarily due to the MCFA in coconut oil that makes it so special and so beneficial. There are only a very few good dietary sources of MCFA. By far the best sources are from coconut and palm kernel oils.

Dr. D'Agostino explains how the Ketogenic Diet can have such a dramatic (and rapid) effect on cancer. All of your body's cells are fueled by glucose. This includes cancer cells. However, cancer cells have one built-in fatal flaw – they do not have the metabolic flexibility of your regular cells and cannot adapt to use ketone bodies for fuel as all your other cells can. So, when you alter your diet and become what's known as "fat-adapted," your body starts using fat for fuel rather than carbs. When you switch out the carbs for healthy fats, you starve the cancer out, as you're no longer supplying the necessary fuel - glucose - for their growth. See page 121

Virgin Coconut Oil, Oil for Life!

Virgin Coconut Oil (VCO) is an oil obtained from the fresh mature kernel of coconut by mechanical or natural means without the use of heat or undergoing chemical refining, bleaching or deodorizing and which does not lead to the alteration of the nature of the oil. It is suitable for consumption without further processing. The active component of Virgin Coconut Oil is **Lauric Acid**, a medium chain fatty acid (MCFA) which is converted to monolaurin in the body that helps boost the immune system and fights microorganisms.

Virgin Coconut Oil is called a "functional food" because of the following health benefits:

- Provides an immediate source of energy.
- Strengthens and supports immune system function.
- It is good for thyroid problems, hypertension, diabetes, allergies.
- Helps prevent bacterial, viral and fungal infections.
- Reduce risk of cancer.
- Aids in promoting weight loss.
- Reduces risk of atherosclerosis and heart disease.
- Improves digestion and nutrient absorption.
- Supplies important nutrients necessary for good health.
- Boosts physical, mental, and emotional wellness.
- Helps prevent or fade stretch marks, scar tissue, & age spots. Helps moisturize your skin, thus prevent premature aging, skin wrinkling. Protects scalp & produce strong silky hair.

Nutrition Facts: Medium Chain Fatty Acids: Lauric Acid 56.9%, Capric Acid 5.5%, Caprylic Acid 5.1%, Long Chain Fatty Acids 29%, Unsaturated Fats 5.7%

Recommended Use: Take 2-3 tablespoons a day before meals. – Coconutresearchcenter.org

Digestion and Nutrient Absorption

For at least five decades researchers have recognized that the Medium Chain Triglycerides (MCT) were digested differently than other fats. This difference has had important applications in the treatment of many digestive and metabolic health conditions and since that time MCT have been routinely used in hospital and baby formulas.

The digestive health advantages of MCT over LCT are due to the differences in the way our bodies metabolize these fats. Because the MCT molecules are smaller, they require less energy and fewer enzymes to break them down for digestion. They are digested and absorbed quickly and with minimal effort.

MCT are broken down almost immediately by enzymes in the saliva and gastric juices so that pancreatic fat-digesting enzymes are not even essential. Therefore, there is less strain on the pancreas and digestive system. This has important implications for patients who suffer from digestive and metabolic problems. Premature and ill infants especially whose digestive organs are underdeveloped, are able to absorb MCT with relative ease, while other fats pass through their systems pretty much undigested. People who suffer from malabsorption problems such as cystic fibrosis, and have difficulty digesting or absorbing fats and fat soluble vitamins, benefit greatly from MCT. They can also be of importance to people suffering from diabetes, obesity, gallbladder disease, pancreatitis Crohn's disease, pancreatic insufficiency, and some forms of cancer.

As we get older our bodies don't function as well as they did in earlier years. The pancreas doesn't make as many digestive enzymes, our intestines don't absorb nutrients as well, the whole process of digestion and elimination moves at a lower rate of efficiency. As a result, older people often suffer from vitamin and mineral deficiencies. Because MCT are easy to digest and improve vitamin and mineral absorption they should be included in the meals of older people. This is easy to do if the meals are prepared with coconut oil.

In the digestive system MCT are broken down into individual fatty acids (MCFA). Unlike other fatty acids, MCFA are absorbed directly from the intestines into the portal vein and sent straight to the liver where they are, for the most part, burned as fuel much like a carbohydrate. In this respect they act more like carbohydrates than like fats.

Other fats require pancreatic enzymes to break them into smaller units. They are then absorbed into the intestinal wall and packaged into bundles of fat (lipid) and protein called lipoproteins. These lipoproteins are carried by the lymphatic system, bypassing the liver, and then dumped into the bloodstream, where they are circulated throughout the body. As they circulate in the blood, their fatty components are distributed to all the tissues of the body. The lipoproteins get smaller and smaller, until there is little left of them. At this time they are picked up by the liver, broken apart, and used to produce energy or, if needed, repackaged into other lipoproteins and sent back into the bloodstream to be distributed throughout the body. Cholesterol, saturated fat, monounsaturated fat, and polyunsaturated fat are all packaged together into lipoproteins and carried throughout the body in this way. In contrast, medium-chain fatty acids are not packaged into lipoproteins but go to the liver where they are converted into energy. Ordinarily they are not stored to any significant degree as body fat. Medium-chain fatty acids produce energy. Other dietary fats produce body fat.

Because of the above advantages, coconut oil has been a lifesaver for many people, particularly the very young and the very old. It is used medicinally in special food preparations for those who suffer digestive disorders and have trouble digesting fats. For the same reason, it is also used in infant formula for the treatment of malnutrition. Since it is rapidly absorbed, it can deliver quick nourishment without putting excessive strain on the digestive and enzyme systems and help conserve the body's energy that would normally be expended in digesting other fats.

Medium-chain triglycerides comprise a major ingredient in most infant formulas commonly used today. See Ketogenic Diet, page 121

Metabolism and Energy

Eating foods containing MCT is like putting high octane fuel into your car. The car runs smoother and gets better gas mileage. Likewise, with MCT your body performs better because it has more energy and greater endurance. Because MCFA are funneled directly to the liver and converted into energy, the body gets a boost of energy. And because MCFA are easily absorbed by the energy-producing organelles of the cells, metabolism increases. This burst of energy has a stimulating effect on the entire body.

The fact that MCT digest immediately to produce energy and stimulate metabolism has led athletes to use them as a means to enhance exercise performance. Studies indicate this may be true. In one study, for example, investigators tested the physical endurance of mice who were given MCT in their daily diet against those that weren't. The study extended over a six-week period. The mice were subjected to a swimming endurance test every other day. They were placed in a pool of water with a constant current. The total swimming time until exhaustion was measured. While at first there was little difference between the groups of mice, those fed MCT quickly began to out-perform the others and continued to improve throughout the testing period. Tests such as this demonstrated that MCT had the ability to enhance endurance and exercise performance, at least in mice.

In another study using humans, conditioned cyclists were used. The cyclists pedaled for three hours. During the last hour they were each given a beverage to drink. Those who received beverages containing MCT out performed the others. Because of studies like these many of the sports drinks and energy bars sold at health food stores contain MCT to provide a quick source of energy.

It's easy to see why athletes would be interested in gaining greater endurance and energy, but what about non- athletes? MCT can do the same for them. If eaten regularly MCT can provide a boost in energy and performance of daily activities. Would you like to increase your energy level throughout the day? If you get tired in the middle of the day or feel you lack energy, adding coconut oil to your daily diet may provide you with a much needed boost to help carry you through. Besides increasing your energy level, there are other very important benefits that results from boosting your metabolic rate: it helps protect you from illness and speeds healing. When metabolism increased, cells function at a higher rate of efficiency. They heal injuries quicker, old and diseased cells are replaced faster, and young, new cells are generated at an increased rate to replace worn-out ones. Even the immune system functions better.

Several health problems such as obesity, heart disease, and osteoporosis are more prevalent in those people who have slow metabolism. Any health condition is made worse if the metabolic rate is slower than normal, because cells can't heal and repair themselves as quickly. Increasing metabolic rate, therefore, provides an increased degree of protection from both degenerative and infectious illnesses. **Source:** Coconut Oil and Medium Chain Triglycerides by Dr. Bruce Fife, The Coconut Oil Miracle

Coronavirus and Virgin Coconut Oil

The corona virus has been reported in at least 23 other countries, including Canada, United States, Australia, France, Japan, Thailand, South Korea, Taiwan, Vietnam, Singapore, Saudi Arabia, and Africa. There have been hundreds of cases reported outside of China, and the numbers are rising. In just over one month the virus has spread worldwide and appears to be blooming into a worldwide pandemic. The World Health Organization has declared a global health emergency. The Chinese government has shut down all travel in and out of Wuhan — a city with a population of 11 million — and the surrounding area in an effort to contain the spread of the disease. Travelers returning home from recently visiting China are being quarantined for at least two weeks.

Coronaviruses (CoV) are a family of RNA (ribonucleic acid) viruses, also called retroviruses. They are called coronaviruses because the virus particle exhibits a characteristic 'corona' (crown) of spiked proteins around its lipid envelope. CoV infections are common in animals and humans. Some strains of CoV are zoonotic, meaning they can be transmitted between animals and humans, but many strains are not.

In humans, CoV can cause symptoms range from those resembling the common cold to deadly, such as Middle East Respiratory Syndrome (caused by MERS-CoV), and Severe Acute Respiratory Syndrome (caused by SARS-CoV).
Patients infected with the new coronavirus, named 2019-nCoV Acute Respiratory Disease (2019-nCoV), usually exhibit severe coughing, which may be accompanied by labored breathing. All cases show radiographic evidence of pneumonia.

Currently, there is no cure or effective medical intervention to treat the virus. The body must fight the infection on its own. Those with weak immune systems, generally the very young and the elderly or those who are in poor health, are most vulnerable. At some point there may be a vaccine developed for it, but that will be a long way off.

Take heart, you are not helpless against this new virus, there is a natural solution that may prove quite useful—coconut oil. The coronavirus is a lipid coated virus, meaning it is encased in a fatty envelope. The medium chain fatty acids in coconut oil, particularly lauric acid, have been shown to kill lipid coated viruses. Coconut oil consists of 63 percent medium chain fatty acids; nearly 50 percent of the oil is lauric acid.

The antiviral action is attributed to solubilizing the lipid envelope of the virus causing it to disintegrate, killing it. In addition, evidence also indicates that lauric acid may interfere with signal transduction in cell replication, preventing the virus from reproducing. All medium chain fatty acids have some antiviral properties; lauric acid is by far the most potent. It is important to note that while MCT oil is composed of 100 percent medium chain fatty acids, it contains no lauric acid, and therefore, would not provide the best protection against the coronavirus. At this time, the daily consumption of coconut oil, at approximately 3 tablespoons (45 ml) per day, might be your best defense.

Dr. Bruce Fife wrote the above article. Doctors Fabian Dayrit, PhD and Mary Newport, MD have co-authored an article on the coronavirus and how it may be possible to treat it using coconut oil and/or monolaurin. You can read *The Potential of Coconut Oil and its Derivatives as Effective and Safe Antiviral Agents Against the Novel Coronavirus (nCoV-2019)*

According to Dr Judy Mikovits, COVID-19 is not caused by SARS-CoV-2 alone, but rather that it's the result of a combination of SARS-CoV-2 and XMRVs (human gammaretroviruses). SARS-CoV-2 also appears to have been manipulated to include components of HIV that destroys immune function along with XMRVs. Those already infected with XMRVs may end up getting serious COVID-19 infection and/or die from the disease. Flu vaccines have spread a host of dangerous viruses around the world, which can then interact with SARS COV-2. Mikovits's research suggests more than 30 million Americans carry XMRVs and other gammaretroviruses in their bodies from contaminated vaccines and blood supply.

Coconut oil with 655 Prime Intranasal Light Therapy (blood oxygenation), LianHua Qingwen capsules and Eight Extraordinary Meridians Qigong are the best immune system boosters to ward off viruses in my international travels. – Ricardo B Serrano

Prevention is better than cure.

Intranasal Light therapy reduces levels of pro-inflammatory cytokines

PBM reduces levels of pro-inflammatory cytokines in activated inflammatory cells.

Intranasal Light Therapy works by reducing the levels of pro-inflammatory cytokines caused by the coronavirus.

Blood storm

Coronaviruses can also cause problems in other systems of the body, due to the hyperactive immune response.

A 2014 study showed that 92 percent of patients with MERS had at least one manifestation of the coronavirus outside of the lungs. In fact, signs of a full body blitz have been witnessed with all three of the zoonotic coronaviruses: elevated liver enzymes, lower white blood cell and platelet count, and low blood pressure. In rare cases, patients have suffered from acute kidney injury and cardiac arrest.

But this isn't necessarily a sign that the virus itself is spreading throughout the body, says Angela Rasmussen, a virologist and associate research scientist at Columbia University Mailman School of Public Health. It might be a cytokine storm.

Cytokines are proteins used by the immune system as alarm beacons—they recruit immune cells to the site of infection. The immune cells then kill off the infected tissue in a bid to save the rest of the body.

Humans rely on our immune systems to keep their cool when facing a threat. But during a runaway coronavirus infection, when the immune system dumps cytokines into the lungs without any regulation, this culling becomes a free-for-all, Rasmussen says "Instead of shooting at a target with a gun, you're using a missile launcher," she says. That's where the problem arises: Your body is not just targeting the infected cells. It is attacking healthy tissue too.

The implications extend outside the lungs. Cytokine storms create inflammation that weakens blood vessels in the lungs and causes fluid to seep through to the air sacs. "Basically you're bleeding out of your blood vessels," Rasmussen says. The storm spills into your circulatory system and creates systemic issues across multiple organs.

From there, things can take a sharp turn for the worse. In some of the most severe COVID-19 cases, the cytokine response—combined with a diminished capacity to pump oxygen to the rest of the body—can result in multi-organ failure. Scientists don't know exactly why some patients experience complications outside of the lung, but it might be linked to underlying conditions like heart disease or diabetes.

"Even if the virus doesn't get to kidneys and liver and spleen and other things, it can have clear downstream effects on all of those processes," Frieman says. And that's when things can get serious. **Credit:** National Geographic article *Here's what coronavirus does to the body (From blood storms to honeycomb lungs) by Amy McKeever and Mechanisms and applications of the anti-inflammatory effects of Photobiomodulation by Michael R Hamblin*
https://www.ncbi.nlm.nih.gov/pmc/articles/PMC5523874/

Can CBD help with Coronavirus Cytokine Storm? In inflammatory states (such as coronavirus cytokine storm), CBD (Cannabidiol) in the form of CBD oil can calm inflammation. Moreover, CBD, but not THC, up-regulates the activation of the STAT3 transcription factor, an element of homeostatic mechanism(s) inducing anti-inflammatory events. See page 19, How Cannabis works; page 95, CBD may be very effective for covid-19

Source: *https://www.hindawi.com/journals/mi/2015/538670/* Evaluation of Serum Cytokines Levels and the Role of Cannabidiol Treatment in Animal Model of Asthma

https://www.ncbi.nlm.nih.gov/pubmed/25356537 Cannabidiol improves lung function and inflammation in mice submitted to LPS-induced acute lung injury.

LLLT acts as cAMP-elevating agent in acute respiratory distress syndrome.

The aim of this work was to investigate if the low-level laser therapy (LLLT) on acute lung inflammation (ALI) induced by lipopolysaccharide (LPS) is linked to tumor necrosis factor (TNF) in alveolar macrophages (AM) from bronchoalveolar lavage fluid (BALF) of mice. LLLT has been reported to actuate positively for relieving the late and early symptoms of airway and lung inflammation. It is not known if the increased TNF mRNA expression and dysfunction of cAMP generation observed in ALI can be influenced by LLLT. For in vivo studies, Balb/c mice (n = 5 for group) received LPS inhalation or TNF intra nasal instillation and 3 h after LPS or TNF-α, leukocytes in BALF were analyzed. LLLT administered perpendicularly to a point in the middle of the dissected bronchi with a wavelength of 660 nm and a dose of 4.5 J/cm(2). The mice were irradiated 15 min after ALI induction. In vitro AM from mice were cultured for analyses of TNF mRNA expression and protein and adenosine3':5'-cyclic monophosphate (cAMP) levels. One hour after LPS, the TNF and cAMP levels in AM were measured by ELISA. RT-PCR was used to measure TNF mRNA in AM. The LLLT was inefficient in potentiating the rolipram effect in presence of a TNF synthesis inhibitor. LLLT attenuated the neutrophil influx and TNF in BALF. In AM, the laser increased the cAMP and reduced the TNF-α mRNA. LLLT increases indirectly the cAMP in AM by a TNF-dependent mechanism.

Source: https://www.ncbi.nlm.nih.gov/pubmed/21184127

Scientists have discovered that light energy (Qi) has positive modulating effects on red blood cells, optimizing their cellular structure and oxygenation capacity. Additionally, photobiomodulation may stimulate mitochondria within white blood cells, potentially leading to an enhanced immune system. Up-regulation of cytochrome c oxidase (CCO) by intranasal light therapy (ILT) can optimize the oxygenation of the blood of ill patients with COVID-19 whose lungs are affected reducing the oxygenation of their blood. ILT also triggers the release of nitric oxide (NO) that inhibits the replication cycle of Severe Acute Respiratory Syndrome Coronavirus.

Source: https://ncbi.nlm.nih.gov/pmc/articles/PMC4971496 and https://jvi.asm.org/content/79/3/1966

According to **Dr. Mikovits**, author of *Plague of Corruption: Restoring Faith in the Promise of Science*, they can't have patents of naturally occurring substances like CBDs, like vitamin C therapies, the natural products, the energy therapies that we could do to stop these coronaviruses. Even *light therapy* would stop the activation of expression… We don't need *vaccines*. We have natural God given immunity, and we know so much about how to develop it in the immune-compromised, how to maintain it.

The Chinese Treatment for COVID-19

"To prevent respiratory diseases caused by virus infections, the Qi deficient immune system has to be strengthened by acupuncture, Qigong, Qi-healing and herbs**.**" – Ricardo B Serrano

Lianhua Qingwen capsules (LQC), which are also used against seasonal influenza, have been part of China's standard of care against COVID-19 since February 2020, and countries like Thailand and Laos have also embraced the product.

LQC, composed of 13 herbs, is said to have "a curative effect in patients with mild symptoms and helps to relieve fever, cough and fatigue," and may also "help prevent the disease from worsening."

Research shows patients who received LQC along with "usual treatment" had improved recovery rates compared to controls (91.5% versus 82.4%). They also recovered faster (seven versus 10 days). *Jinhua Qinggan* granules are also part of China's standard therapies list for COVID-19. *Jinhua Qinggan* granules contain a mix of 12 different herbs, including licorice, mint and honeysuckle.

A compound found in licorice root called *liquiritin* appears to prevent SARS-CoV-2 reproduction and inhibit proinflammatory cytokines. It also has anti-inflammatory and neuroprotective properties, modulates the immune system and helps improve lung function.

Source: https://www.ncbi.nlm.nih.gov/pmc/articles/PMC7229744/ Efficacy and safety of *Lianhua qingwen* capsules, a repurposed Chinese herb, in patients with coronavirus disease 2019: A multicenter, prospective, randomized controlled trial

Glossary of Terms

Amino acid; the building block of proteins; there are over 20 different amino acids present in nature.

Antioxidant; any one of a large group of natural or synthetic substances whose presence slows down the deterioration induced by oxygen of other substances such as fatty acids.

Cell membrane; a double layer of fatty material (phosphatides) and proteins which surrounds each living cell of all organisms.

Cholesterol: a complex fatty substance which has many important functions in the body. It can be made in the body or supplied through foods of animal origin. Excess cholesterol may be deposited in artery linings.

Complex carbohydrate; sugar molecules linked together in various ways to make digestible molecules such as starch and glycogen or indigestible molecules of fiber which include cellulose, bran, pectin, lignin, mucilage and gum.

Deficiency disease; the effect on health of shortage or lack of any one or more of the 45 or so essential nutrients. **Degenerative disease**: loss of capacity of cells, tissues and organs to function normally. Causes include deficiency of essential nutrients, presence of interfering substances, excess of substances or imbalance in the relative concentrations of substances.

Eicosapentaenoic acid (EPA 20:5w3): a 20 carbon fatty acid with 5 double bonds in its chain. It is found in high concentrations in cold-water fish and marine animals, and also in retina, brain, adrenals and testes. It can be manufactured in healthy human tissue from the essential linolenic acid (18:3w3).

Enzyme: a protein produced by the body to catalyze (facilitate) particular chemical reactions. The enzyme which catalyzes the reaction is not itself changed thereby.

Essential amino acid: any one of 8 amino acids which the body requires but cannot manufacture and must therefore be obtained from foods.

Essential fatty acid: either of 2 fatty acids which the body requires, cannot make from other substances and which must therefore be supplied by the food. The names of these 2 are linoleic acid (18:2w6) and linolenic acid(18:3w3). **Essential fatty acid deficiency**: shortage of one of both of the essential fatty acids and the attendant effects on health of this shortage.

Essential nutrient: any one of about 45 different substances that are known to be necessary for body structure and physical health. About 20 minerals, 15 vitamins, 8 amino acids and 2 essential fatty acids must come from the foods we eat, since the body cannot manufacture them out of other substances.

Evening primrose: a weed whose seeds contain within them the essential linoleic acid (18:2w6) and also a product made from it, known as gammalinolenic acid.

Fat: three fatty acids hooked to a glycerol molecule in an ester linkage. In common usage, it refers to those substances that fit the above description and are hard at temperature because they contain mostly saturated fatty acids. Fatty acid: a carbon chain with an organic acid group at one end, and hydrogens attached to the rest of the carbon atoms in the chain. The chain length can vary from 4 to 26 or more. Fatty degeneration: fatty deposits which interfere with normal biological functions, commonly found in arteries, around tumors, in liver, and other internal organs.

Flax: a plant whose seed oil contains both essential fatty acids in large quantities especially the more rare linolenic acid (18:3w3). It also contains many other essential nutrients, as well as mucilage and fiber, which aid the body in the elimination of excess cholesterol, and help to prevent the reabsorption of toxic wastes from the large intestine.

Free radical: a molecule or molecular fragment with a single or unpaired electron which, wanting to be paired, steals electrons from other pairs. Free radical reactions occur normally in biological processes.

Gammalinolenic acid: a substance made from the essential linoleic acid (18:2w6) by healthy cells, also found in mother's milk and evening primrose oil. It is used therapeutically in several combinations in which the body's ability to make it from linoleic acid is impaired.

Glycogen: glucose molecules hooked together in long chains and stored in the liver and muscle of animals as energy reserves. It is also called animal starch.

High density lipoprotein (HDL): one of the vehicles found in the blood stream, which carries fats and cholesterol. It is the good type of cholesterol, which returns excess cholesterol from the cells to the liver, where it is changed into bile acids and poured into the intestine to aid in fat digestion on its way out of the body.

Hydrogenation: a commercial process by which oils are turned into fats, by destroying the double bonds in the fatty acids and saturating the carbon atoms with hydrogen.

Krebs cycle: the body's main way of releasing the energy stored in the chemical bonds available for the body's requirements. Carbohydrates are its main fuel, but fats and proteins may also be used. It is also called the tricarboxylic acid cycle and the citric acid cycle.

Lecithin: a nutritional substance containing fatty acids, glycerol, phosphate groups and choline. Its health value resides in its content of essential fatty acids and choline. Soybeans are a good source of lecithin which contains both essential fatty acids. Lecithin is part of the structure of the membranes of cells and organelles.

Linoleic acid (LA 18:2w6): an 18 carbon fatty acid with 2 double bonds, positioned between w carbon atoms 6 and 7, and 9 and 10. It is one of the 2 essential fatty acids. The body cannot make it, requires it for life, and must therefore obtain from food. It is sensitive to destruction by light, oxygen and high temperatures, and extremely important to the body's health. Its absence is fatal. Deficiency causes severe problems in every cell, tissue, and organ. The body makes several other important substances from it.

Linolenic acid (LNA 18:3w3): an 18 carbon fatty acid with 3 double bonds, positioned between w carbons 3 and 4, 6 and 7, and 9 and 10. It is the second of the 2 essential fatty acids. The body cannot make it, requires it for life, and must therefore obtain it from food. It is extremely sensitive to destruction by light, oxygen, and high temperature. Its absence is fatal. Deficiency is linked to degenerative disease. Modern diets contain only 1/5 as much of this essential substance as traditional diets.

Lipid: the chemist's collective name for fats, oils and other fatty substances. Lipoprotein: fatty substances (fats, oils, phosphatides and cholesterol) associated with protein materials. Specifically, it refers to transport vehicles for fats and cholesterol in the blood and lymph.

Low density lipoprotein: vehicles which transport fats and cholesterol via the blood stream to the cells. An excess of these vehicles is associated with cardiovascular disease; hence it is also called the bad cholesterol.

Metabolism: all of the chemical changes that take place in the body that make physical life possible.

Medium Chain Fatty Acid: based on molecular size or length of the carbon chain in the fatty acid, also called Medium Chain Triglycerides found in coconut oil. Monounsaturated fatty acid (MUFA): a fatty acid which contains one double bond between carbon atoms somewhere in the fatty chain found in olive oil.

Orthomolecular: literally, of the right molecules. In nutrition, it is the maintenance of health and the treatment of disease by varying the concentrations of substances normally present in the body (vitamins, minerals, fatty acids, amino acids, enzymes, hormones)

Oxidize: the addition of oxygen, subtraction of hydrogen, or addition of electrons to a substance, usually accompanied by a release of energy.

Phosphatide: also called phospholipid; a class of fatty compounds found in membranes, consisting of 2 fatty acid molecules, a glycerol molecule, a phosphate group, and some other groups hooked to the phosphate. Lecithin is the most famous example.

Prostaglandin: a fatty acid partially oxidized in a very specific and controlled way by enzymes made in the body for just this purpose. Prostaglandins have hormone-like functions in the regulation of cell activity. There are about 30 different prostaglandins known so far.

Protein: a group of complex molecules with specific and precise structural and chemical functions. They are made by linking together amino acids (over 20 different kinds of amino acids are known) in a specific linear sequence and then folding these chains in particular 3-dimensional ways. Enzymes, muscle and egg white are examples of protein.

Saturated fatty acid: a fatty acid with no double bonds in the carbon chain, and with every possible position on the carbon atoms taken up by hydrogen atoms.

Simple carbohydrate: a simple sugar. Glucose, fructose and lactose are examples. Simple carbohydrates are absorbed into the blood stream rapidly; excess consumption may lead to hypoglycemia, diabetes and cardiovascular problems, as well as obesity.

Trans-fatty acid: a fatty in which the hydrogen atoms on the carbon atoms involved in a double bond are situated on opposite sides of the fatty chain. Triglyceride: a molecule of fat or oil. It consists of 3 fatty acid molecules hooked to glycerol backbone. This is the form in which fatty acids are stored in the body's fat tissues and in the seeds of plants. Unsaturated fatty acid: a fatty acid with one or more double bonds between carbons in its chain.

Source: Fats and Oils by Udo Erasmus, 1986.

Herbs for Cancer – Essiac, Pau d'arco, Chaparral, Guyabano, Turmeric and Cannabis Hemp Oil

Essiac

Essiac, a harmless herbal tea, was used by Canadian nurse Rene Caisse to successfully treat thousands of cancer patients from 1920s until her death in 1978 at the age of ninety. Refusing payment for her services, instead accepting only voluntary contributions, the Bracebridge, Ontario, nurse brought remissions to hundreds of documented cases, many abandoned as "hopeless" or "terminal" by orthodox medicine. She aided countless more in prolonging life and relieving pain. Caisse obtained remarkable results against a wide variety of cancers, treating persons by administering Essiac through hypodermic injections or oral ingestion.

The formula for the herbal remedy was given to Caisse in 1922 by a hospital patient whose breast cancer had been healed by an Ontario Indian medicine man.

The principal herbs in Essiac include burdock root, turkey rhubarb root (Indian rhubarb), sheep sorrel, and slippery elm bark. Burdock root, a key active ingredient, is also a major ingredient of the Hoxsey herbal remedy. Two Hungarian scientists in 1996 reported "considerable antitumor activity" in a purified fraction of burdock. In addition, as also discussed, scientists at Nagoya University, in 1984 discovered burdock contains a new type of desmutagen, a substance uniquely capable of reducing cell mutation either in the absence or in the presence of metabolic activation. So important is this property, the Japanese researchers named it the B-factor, for "burdock factor." Another herb in Essiac, turkey rhubarb root, was demonstrated to have antitumor activity in the sarcoma-37 animal test system. Herbalists, however, believe that the synergistic interaction of herbal ingredients contributes to their therapeutic effects. They point out that laboratory tests on a single, isolated compound from one herbal formula fail to address this synergistic potency.

The Canadian herbal remedy developed by Rene Caisse is not being recommended in this chapter as a "magic bullet" for all cancers. There is no hard evidence on what percentage of Caisse's patients survived five years or more. Nor is there any reliable statistical evidence on the efficacy of contemporary Essiac or Essiac-like herbal formulas (*Cessiac and Yuccalive herbal formulas*). Despite the dramatic, near-miraculous cures Caisse undoubtedly achieved, an unknown percentage of patients under her care succumbed to their disease, perhaps too severely ill to be treated.

The world has become an infinitely more polluted place since the 1920s and '30s, when Caisse did her pioneering work. Carcinogenic, toxic chemicals and radioactive isotopes that pollute our water, air, and food also reside permanently in the cells of our bodies, weakening our natural immunity and possibly making the remission of cancer more difficult. For these reasons, combining Essiac with nutritional and other approaches may make the most sense. **Risk Information**: Do not take with MAO inhibitor medications and other medications.

Pau d'Arco

Pau d'Arco is a popular herbal remedy for cancer sold in health food stores. Available in the form of tea bags as well as capsules and loose powder, it is also known as lapacho, ipe roxo, and taheebo. The herbal tea is prepared from the inner bark of various species of a large South American tree that flowers a vibrant pink, purple, or yellow. This tree is the Tabebuia tree, native to Brazil and Argentina.

In South America, pau d'arco is widely used as a treatment for cancer and illnesses such as colds, flus, fevers, malaria, infections, syphilis, gonorrhea, and at least one kind of lupus. The tree also grows in India, where it is used for similar complaints. Supporters of pau d'arco say that it builds up immunity to disease, combat infection, and eliminates pain and inflammation. According to the late Jonathan Hartwell - biochemist, researcher for the National Cancer Institute, and author of the definitive *Plants Used Against Cancer* - pau d'arco tea has been used in folk remedies for cancers of the pancreas, esophagus, intestines, head, lung, prostate, and tongue; Hodgkin's disease; leukemia; and lupus erythematosus. One species of Tabebuia, T. serratofolia, is traditionally used in Colombia to treat cancer.

In the United States, word-of-mouth reports and written testimonials from cancer patients link tumor regression or remission to drinking pau d'arco tea.

Bill Wead, whose 1985 book, *Second Opinion*, focuses on pau d'arco as a cancer treatment, had on file "literally hundreds of testimonies as to the efficacy of Lapacho." His book presents a number of case histories of cancer patients who attribute their recovery to the herbal medication.

However, "there is very strong evidence that once remission has occurred, it is necessary to continue drinking the tea," according to Wead.

He observed that in "a few" cases where remission had occurred after drinking pau d'arco, the cancer later returned. In some of these cases, the recurrence came only after the person stopped drinking the tea. Wead also emphasized that pau d'arco does not work for everyone. There is no reliable statistical data on pau d'arco's efficacy against cancer or on its long term effects, positive or negative. But an impressive body of laboratory evidence plus a handful of clinical studies indicate that lapachol, an organic compound present in the tea, has strong antitumor properties as well as antibiotic and antimalarial action.

Here is a brief summary of a few of the studies done on pau d'arco worldwide:

- Nine patients were given oral doses of lapachol for twenty to sixty days or longer. One complete tumor regression and two partial tumor regressions occurred. One patient had hepatic adenocarcinoma; another had basal cell carcinoma of the cheek with metastases to the cervix, and the third had ulcerated squamous cell carcinoma of the oral cavity.
- The life span of leukemia mice treated with a lapachol derivative for nine days increased 80 percent over a control group.
- West German scientists investigating pau d'arco for antitumor effects found that nine constituent compounds have dose-dependent immunomodulating effects on human immune system cells. This suggests that the ability of pau d'arco compounds to destroy cancer cells may be at least partly due to stimulation of the immune system.
- Extracts of pau d'arco (rather than lapachol alone) killed cancer cells in culture and reduced the occurrence of lung metastases in mice following surgery to remove tumors. Five times as many mice survived in the group given pau d'arco compared with the control group.
- Lapachol was shown to have significant activity against Walker 256 carcinoma, especially when administered orally to animals implanted with this tumor.
- Lapachol was found to be an excellent antitumor agent and antibiotic.

Bill Wead has the following guidelines concerning pau d'arco:

- Do not boil the tea in a tin pot or kettle. Ideally, a glass pot should be used. Stainless steel is acceptable.
- The packaging material of the tea should not be made of plastic.
- Pau d'arco in pill form is of little or no value.

Wayne Martin claims that if all cancer patients at an early stage of their disease practiced self-medication with pau d'arco tea, the cancer death rate would greatly decline. He says that the action of pau d'arco appears to be similar to that of warfarin sodium, an anticoagulant drug. (An anticoagulant is a substance that delays or prevents the clotting of blood.)

Warfarin sodium has been used in treating advanced cancer with some success. Clinical trials suggest that oral warfarin sodium has the ability to slow down tumor growth rate. According to this line of thinking, warfarin-like anticoagulants inhibit the formation of *fibrin,* the protein coat that surrounds and protects malignant tumors. *Fibrin* is believed to induce *angiogenesis*, the development of a vascular network providing blood and nourishment to a new cancer colony. In the Winter-Spring 1991 issue of *Cancer Victors Journal*, Martin reviews a number of experimental and clinical studies suggesting that warfarin-like drugs help prevent cancer from metastasizing. He speculates that pau d'arco also has this action.

Risk Information: Should not be taken with aspirin, ticlopidine, gingko biloba, ginseng, warfarin & heparin, and pregnant or breastfeeding mother. Should not be taken with MAO inhibitor medications and other medications.

Chaparral

Native Americans, for centuries, have brewed the stems and leaves of chaparral to treat cancer, venereal disease, arthritis, rheumatism, tuberculosis, colds, stomach disorders, and skin infections. In folk medicine, chaparral has been used for leukemia and cancers of the kidney, liver, lung, and stomach, and for AIDS.

Besides containing immune-stimulating polysaccharides, chaparral has a key ingredient *nor-dihydroguaiaretic acid* (NDGA), which has been shown to have powerful antitumor properties. NDGA inhibits electron transport in the *mitochondria*, or "energy-producing factories," within cancer cells, thereby depriving tumors of the electrical energy they require to exist.

NDGA is also a potent inhibitor of *glycolysis*, the breakdown of sugars and other carbohydrates by enzymes. The work of Nobel Prize-winning biochemist Otto Warburg indicates that cancer cells live by fermenting sugar in anaerobic (airless) reactions. NDGA is a strong inhibitor of both anaerobic and aerobic glycolysis. Dean Burk, PhD, outlined a possible mechanism of action for NDGA based on Warburg's work, suggesting that chaparral may actually reorient the fermentation process of cancer cells. Burk performed experiments with NDGA at the National Cancer Institute. His research showed that in laboratory cultures, "this is a very active agent against cancer," in the words of Dr. Charles Smart of the University of Utah Medical Center.

Modern science lends support to the Indians' faith in the healing virtues of chaparral. To a curious visitor, a Pima Indian of Arizona once said, "This plant cures everything. It is what nature gave us." The Mexicans call the creosote bush *gobernadora* ("governess") because chaparral reputedly governs the body, reversing all manner of ailments. This belief in chaparral's therapeutic powers is shared by many Native American tribes, who use the herb to treat everything from the common cold to bladder stones to cancer. Chaparral is recognized in current herbal medicine as "one of the best herbal antibiotics, being useful against bacteria, viruses, and parasites," writes naturopath Michael Tierra in *The Way of Herbs*.

Until 1967, NDGA was a common additive in baking mixes, candies, oils, lards, frozen foods, vitamins, and various pharmaceuticals. An antioxidant, it kept these items from spoiling by preventing the growth of bacteria. It is a powerful scavenger of free radicals, the reactive chemicals that form continuously in the body and have been shown to damage cells.

Tom Murdock, founder of *Nature's Way*, a well-known herb company, reported that chaparral helped his wife's breast cancer go into remission when conventional medical treatment failed. After Lavoli Murdock's recovery, Tom began selling the desert shrub; chaparral thus helped start the family's herbal business.

A formula for chaparral tea as a cancer remedy is given by Arlin J. Brown in *March of Truth on Cancer*. Brown's recipe is as follows; Put 4 ounces in a 2-quart bottle and add 1 cup of boiling water. Steep for about 10 minutes and then fill to about 1 inch from the top with boiling water. Put on tight-fitting lid, set in the sun for 2 days, and strain. Drink 3 cups a day.

Brown, who runs the Arlin J. Brown Information Center dispensing information on alternative cancer therapies, advises that patients who drink chaparral should take a good iron supplement. "If you take chaparral for a few years without iron supplement, it will destroy the blood-forming organs in the body," he says. Laboratory tests and clinical experience with the desert herb indicate that it is nontoxic, generally has no side effects, and is compatible with medication.

Even though there are cases of people who brought their cancer into remission on chaparral alone, Brown strongly advises against such a regimen. "To take only chaparral tea, or pau d'arco, or Essiac, or whatever is not enough. A person with cancer needs an intensive program combining detoxification and immune enhancement. Chaparral taken alone might help in some early cases of cancer, but it's by no means a total therapy. You need to detoxify the body - through vegetable and fruit juices, herbs, blood purifiers, and other measures such as colonic irrigations or coffee enemas. Then you need immune enhancement by going on a proper diet and immune-boosting supplements. Only through such a program can cancer patients maximize their chances of preventing a recurrence."

Herbalist Michael Tierra has outlined a therapeutic anticancer program combining diet and detoxification. In *The Way of Herbs*, Tierra specifies an herbal formula that he believes can aid the body in detoxifying itself. This formula emphasizes "the most powerful blood purifiers in the herbal kingdom," chaparral and echinacea, and also includes red clover blossoms, cascara sagrada, astragalus, ginseng, and other herbs. Another anticancer formula featuring chaparral, echinacea root, pau d'arco, and red clover blossoms is given in Tierra's *Planetary Herbology*, which attempts to synthesize Western herbal medicine and traditional Chinese and Ayurvedic systems. Recognizing that cancers and tumors are "difficult to treat," Tierra sets forth a balanced diet for the cancer patient based on whole grains, beans, and fresh vegetables, and excluding red meat and (usually) dairy foods.

Another variation on chaparral therapy is Jason Winters Herbal Tea. Jason Winters, a former stunt man, reportedly healed himself of terminal cancer after cobalt treatments failed to reduce the size of a large tumor on his neck. He claims to have eliminated the tumor himself in three weeks by drinking a tea made from chaparral, red clover (a principal ingredient of Hoxsey herbs), and the root of a certain white flower from Singapore that he dubbed herbaline. Winters has never divulged the identity of this flower, supposedly because if he did, the plant might soon become very scarce.

Scientific research on chaparral has continued sporadically. Recent studies by microbiologist Emiliano Mora at Auburn University have demonstrated that an extract of chaparral kills malignant cancer cells in test tubes. In experiments dating back to the 1960s, NDGA had significant growth-inhibiting activity against some animal tumors, though not against others. Despite the intriguing results obtained with chaparral in the laboratory and the known cases of cancer remission, the resourceful desert shrub remains condemned on the American Cancer Society's Unproven Methods blacklist. But chaparral, an incredibly adaptive plant, may outlive even the ACS's condemnation. **Risk Information**: Should not be taken with MAO inhibitor medications and other medications. **Source**: Options, the Alternative Cancer Therapy Book by Richard Walters, 1993. Pp. 105-118, 128-134, 135-140.

Guyabano (Soursop, Graviola), Herbal Medicine and Its Health Benefits

Guyabano tree, or soursop in English (Scientific Name : Anona muricata Linn.) is a small tree, usually about 5 to 7 meters high. Guyabano is a fruit bearing tree, broadleaf, flowering, and evergreen that is native to Central America, the Caribbean and South America. Guyabano can be found in Mexico, Colombia, Brazil, Peru, and

Venezuela. Guyabano or Soursop are also native in sub-Saharan African countries. Guyabano or Soursop is adaptable to tropical climate and are currently cultivated for its fruit in Malaysia, Indonesia and Philippines.

Guyabano and Cancer Guyabano or soursop is also known to possess medicinal properties that include cancer fighting activity. In a study published in the "Journal of Medicinal Chemistry", fourteen structurally diverse *Annonaceous acetogenins*, found in Guyabano extract were identified and tested for their ability to inhibit the growth of adriamycin resistant human mammary adenocarcinoma cells. This cell line is known to be multidrug resistant cancer cells. Some of the *acetogenins* from the guyabano extract were found to be more potent than *adriamycin* and thus may have chemotherapeutic potential, especially with regard to multidrug resistant tumors.. Since 1976, the National Cancer Institute found that Guyabano's "leaves and stems" were found effective in attacking and destroying malignant cells but was never released to the public. Further studies found that Guyabano attacks only cancer cells, not healthy cells.

Guyabano and Diabetes An article in "African Journal of Traditional Complementary and Alternative Medicine" about in 2008 have reported that a clinical study done on rats induced with diabetes mellitus then fed with guyabano (Annona Muricata Linn) extracts showed positive effects of lowering the blood sugar levels in animals. Another study reported by the same publication showed that animals with induced diabetes mellitus that consumed guyabano extract has showed remarkable increase of antioxidants in their blood and that there is less liver damage. The findings of this laboratory animal study suggest that (guyabano) Annona muricata extract has a protective, beneficial effect on hepatic tissues subjected to STZ-induced oxidative stress, possibly by decreasing lipid peroxidation and indirectly enhancing production of insulin and endogenous antioxidants. Although the reports suggested that guyabano extracts have promising medicinal benefits for diabetes mellitus. There is no sufficient study done on its effects to humans with diabetes.

Guyabano and Inflammation In a report that was published in "International Journal of Molecular Sciences" dated 2010, Antinociceptive and anti-inflammatory activities of the ethanol extract from guyabano leaves (Annona muricata Linn) were investigated in animal models.. In a chemically induced edema to the paw of rats showed that the guyabano ethanol extract has significantly reduced the exudate volume. These results suggest that Annona muricata can be an active source of substances with antinociceptive and anti-inflammatory activities.

Guyabano and Herpes Simplex Virus A study published in "Journal of Ethnopharmacology", 1mg/ml of ethanol extract of Annona muricata (Annonaceae, Guyabano) in Petunia nyctaginiflora (Solanaceae) aqueous extract can inhibit the activity of Herpes simplex virus-1 (HSV-1).

Guyabano and Depression In a study published in the "Journal of Pharmacy and Pharmacology", extracts from the fruit and the leaves of Guyabano (Annona muricata - Annonaceae) contains three alkaloids, annonaine (1), nornuciferine (2) and asimilobine (3), that upon tests have shown to inhibit binding of [3H]rauwolscine to 5-HTergic 5-HT1A receptors in calf hippocampus. These results imply that Guyabano fruit (Annona muricata) possesses anti-depressive effects.

Guyabano and Antibacterial Effects In a report published in "Revista do Instituto de Medicina Tropical de São Paulo", a study has been made to determine the antibacterial effects of aqueous and ethanolic extracts of seeds of moringa (Moringa oleifera) and pods of guyabano (Annona muricata). The aqueous extracts of guyabano (annona muricata) showed an antibacterial effect against Staph aureus and Vibrio cholerae, but the antibacterial activity by the ethanol extracts of this plant was not demonstrated. **Risk Information**: Should not be taken if you have any neurodenegerative disorders, Parkinson's disease, or taking antihypertensive or MAO inhibitor medications. Source: rain-tree.com, medicalhealthguide.com/herb/guyabano.htm and hsionline.com

"Coconut oil, CBD oil, intranasal light therapy, LianHua Qingwen capsules and Qigong are the best immune system boosters to ward off COVID- 19. There are better safer therapies than vaccines to treat COVID-19." - Ricardo B Serrano

CBD may be very effective for covid-19 for several reasons.

- Enhancing the endocannabinoid system and regulating ACE2.
- Inhibiting inflammatory cytokines. (IL-6, TNFa, NF-kB) promoting IL10 (anti-inflammatory)
- Preventing cellular oxidative stress. inhibiting reactive oxygen and reactive nitrosative species. Promoting Glutathione & superoxide dismutase enzyme production.
- Inhibiting TLR4 (an intracellular signaling pathway NF-kB and inflammatory cytokine production which is responsible for activating the innate immune system).
- Inhibiting adenosine A2A receptor that regulates glutamate and dopamine release.
- Preventing hypoxic injury of brain, lung, and cardiac tissue.
- Compliment antibiotic therapy by preventing bacterial resistance.
- Stabilize permeability of membranes in lung.
- Inhibit immune cell migration into lung.
- Inhibiting exosome/microvesicle release of virions from infected cells (seen in cancer) and activation of virion proteins through anti-oxidation pathways.
- Inhibits 5HT(1A) stress response influencing the survival and death of WBC, migration and platelet aggregation.

Recent warnings about the use of anti-inflammatory drugs including corticosteroids in common viral disease is appropriate. Inflammation and fever are normal responses that stimulate healing. But in some patients the inflammation cannot be controlled and leads to severe acute respiratory syndrome (SARS) through acute lung injury (ALI). Inflammation reduction is only one aspect of multiple ways that CBD has to limit Covid-19 illness. Cannabinoids may inhibit attachments points for virus (SARS-angiotensin II Receptors), immuno-regulate mast cell, induce TH2 shifts (resolving inflammation), reduce numbers of macrophage/monocytes, inhibit inflammatory cell migration, inhibit inflammatory cytokines (IL-1,2,6,17), inhibit oxidative stress (intracellular), shift into repair mode anabolic (vs breakdown mode catabolic metabolism) and stimulate mitochondria regeneration, energy production and proliferation (doi:10.1016/j.mehy.2019.109371), block acute lung injury TLR4 receptors (doi: 10.1016/j.cell.2008.02.043) and A(2A) adenosine receptors (doi: 10.1016/j.ejphar.2011.12.043), relax smooth muscles of respiratory airways, inhibit apoptosis of respiratory cells. All of this occurs with the side benefits of pain control without reparatory depression (as seen with opioids). - Dr. Philip Blair

COVID-19 causes ARDS (Acute Respiratory Disease Syndrome)

ARDS is a clinical syndrome with high mortality rate and incidence of 4.5-7.1% of all patients admitted to intensive care units. In the lung, omega-3 fatty acid could reduce the number of leuckocytes, and permeability of alveolar capillary membrane, and production of proinflammatory cytokines like interleukin 6, 8 and TNFa. In this study of 58 ICU patients with ARDS use of 720mg omega-3 gel caps three times per day decreased the mortality by 87%. Importantly, omega-3 replaced omega-6 and -9 fats. Omega-3 achieve this effect by conversion to endocannabinoids signalling the immune system to block inflammation. (Anti-inflammatory w-3 endocannabinoid epoxides, doi/10.1073/pnas.1610325114). Cannabidiol also activates a similar anti-inflammatory, endocannabinoid cascade. *Source: https://www.ncbi.nlm.nih.gov/pmc/articles/PMC4312405/* The Effect of Omega-3 Fatty Acids on ARDS: A Randomized Double-Blind Study

To avoid adverse effects, **CBD** oil should not be taken together with intranasal light therapy. Intranasal light therapy like X-Plus is applied by itself every two days or with CBD oil taken in-between. See Can CBD help with COVID-19 Cytokine Storm?, page 85

CBD inhibits cancer cell growth; neuro-protective; promotes bone growth; reduces seizures, blood sugar levels, function of the immune system, inflammation, risk of artery blockage, small intestine contractions, vomiting and nausea; relieves pain and anxiety; slows bacterial growth and antibacterial; suppresses muscle spasms; tranquilizing; treats psoriasis; vasorelaxant.

Turmeric (Curcumin) and Cannabis Hemp Oil

In Sri Lanka with low cancer rate population, a typical diet includes large amounts of turmeric root (Curcuma longa) – a spice that contains curcumin, used in curry powders. And Dr. Ralph W. Moss, PhD listed the following as three of the key benefits of curcumin intake:

1. Rich in antioxidants
2. A natural anti-inflammatory
3. Inhibits growth of new blood vessels in tumors (*angiogenesis*)

It seems that the citizens of Sri Lanka are centuries ahead of the Western world in taking advantage of the cancer-fighting benefits of curcumin, an *angiogenesis* inhibitor.

You can add it to soups, chilis, casseroles, stir-fry, and nearly anything complimented by a smoky, earthy flavor. You can sprinkle it on eggs or use it in a marinade, rub or drink it as tea or in pill form. Turmeric is best mixed with pepper to bring out its key benefits.

Green tea, another angiogenesis inhibitor, should be taken with turmeric to potentiate its benefits.

Risk information: Curcumin should not be taken with anti-coagulant medications or anti-inflammatory drugs. **Source:** Health Sciences Institute (hsionline.com)

Cannabis CBD hemp oil is another angiogenesis inhibitor which should not be taken with hypertensive, antidiabetic and anti-inflammatory drugs together with chemotherapy, radiation for cancer treatment.

Anti-cancer properties of Cannabis CBD hemp oil: Anti-proliferative - prevents cancer cells from reproducing; anti-metastatic - stops cancer from spreading; apoptotic - induces cancer cells to commit suicide; and anti-angiogenic effect - inhibits growth of new blood vessels in tumors (angiogenesis).

Cannabis does not affect disease as much as it affects the endocannabinoid system (ECS) that regulates the processes affecting said inflammatory related diseases. Proper activation of the ECS helps to homeostatically regulate the inflammation in the body that is associated with many diseases.

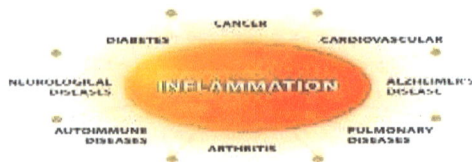

Reference: How Medical Cannabis Works, page19; Holistic Biochemistry of Cannabinoids, page 20; Endocannabinoid Deficiency, page112; Wei Qi Field in Medical Qigong, page 113; Final Notes, page 134

Herbs and Qigong for Healing Cancer

Does it imply that if a cancer patient take herbs and practice Qigong diligently, he or she can be cured of cancer?
The following write-up will provide the answer.

One of the founders of the Cancer Recovery Society in China, told this story during a lecture about the use of Qigong for recovery from cancer and other diseases:

"When people are diagnosed with a life-threatening disease they are often exhausted in body, mind, and spirit. It is as if they are forced to crawl slowly and begin to think of their world as a terribly limited place and their experience of life as scary and depressing. I liken this to the body level of the Three Treasures – Jing, Qi and Shen, the stage of the caterpillar. At this level we are simply looking for a way to survive. We focus on the body, the most limited aspect of ourselves. When we start to do Qigong (and take herbs) we begin to change because we get a sense that our self is not limited. The simple practice of Qigong (and taking herbs) begins a process in the body that is wonderfully healing. The pressure of the experience of the disease plus the support of Qigong friends creates the permission to take on the challenge of becoming a new person.

The caterpillar uses the Qi to spin a cocoon. In our group work with Qigong (and taking herbs) we use the building up of the Qi to create the safety and courage to be reborn. This is our cocoon. We meet to do our practice of Qigong and we have tea and discussion afterward that we call social oncology. You know that when the caterpillar is in the cocoon, its former self is transformed to a new being. In our process of recovery from disease, we often explore uncomfortable things about our lives, talk about things we have kept hidden, and improve our sense of humor. Through this transformational process we create a new self. Just as the caterpillar constructs a cocoon to become a butterfly.

Eventually, we emerge with wings to fly. Many in the Qigong groups recover their health and are reborn as new people who have a completely different attitude about life. Some of our members do not recover but through the Qigong process and group support they become butterflies too, and fly free in a different way. The goal in our work is not just to cure diseases, but to heal. Sometimes healing does not accomplish a cure. But still the person is like a butterfly because he or she has the love of the Qigong group to support a needed transformation. Through Qigong and the love and support of our friends, we gain the courage to transform from a caterpillar, to enter the cocoon and be liberated as a butterfly."

The best answer for what to expect in Qigong (and taking herbs) is to have no expectations. If your mind is crowded with expectations, it cannot be free to perceive what else is really there. In reality, one can learn Qigong from a mentor who is someone who agrees to foster your growth and learning.

Most forms of Qigong have a broad range of benefits and it is through regular practice that one will gain from it. When you discover the Qi, watch it, and cultivate it, let it teach you and you will learn something everyday. Just like sunflowers that come from one seed and create hundreds of seeds that then create hundreds of sunflowers that create thousands of seeds - through your expanded awareness and your practice, your Yuan Qi will multiply.

The eight extraordinary channels are one of the most fascinating aspects of the acupuncture channel system. These channels are the bridge between prenatal and postnatal influences in our life. The eight extraordinary channel's terrain is Jing, essence, and source Qi. These channels influence the yuan, or deep layers of our body, mind and spirit.

The pathways of the eight extraordinary meridians are rooted in the Lower Dantian / Mingmen.

*With thanks to Master Zhao Ji Feng, the President of Guolin Qigong Research Centre in Qingdao, Shandong, China, author of Guolin Qigong training manual and an intestinal cancer survivor. See Guo Lin New Qigong, page 56; Reishi Mushroom, page 63; Guo Lin Qigong and Tonic Herbs, page 68; and Get Well Verse for Cancer Patients, page 112

CONCLUSION

Dr. Joseph Gold said, "Effective cancer control may lie, rather, with therapy of the 'shift' to glycolysis, than with tumor therapy, potentially obviating such developments as drug resistance and major drug toxicity. It is here theorized that *cancer* is a *normal process* invoked by the body as a protective device against tissue damage, senescence and death. It is the most exquisite of paradoxes that the more the body calls upon glycolysis to combat oxidative stress, the more likely it is that the body's protective mechanism will lead to its almost certain confrontation with death."

Hopefully, I have answered in this book the important scientific theory on what cancer is, why cachexia is the condition that kills most people with cancer, the dosages of Hydrazine Sulfate, an anti-cachexia agent, recommended by Dr. Joseph Gold, the contraindications regarding the avoidance of alcohol, barbiturates or tranquilizers, pain killers and tyramine-rich foods.

These important contraindications are not only for your safety but also because the success of the hydrazine sulfate therapy depends on it.

Consultation is a must with a medical doctor regarding diagnostic examination for cancer such as laboratory tests, and drug consultation you should avoid such as painkillers, barbiturates or tranquilizers. Alternative Oriental treatments such as herbs, acupuncture, acupressure and Qigong should act as substitutes for the painkillers, and tranquilizers or barbiturates the patient maybe taking.

Alkaline ionized water with supplements such as Cessiac tea, green tea, Reishi mushrooms, Kerson Fruit or Muntingia calabura (aratiles), Budwig diet with *Turmeric, and oils such as flax seed oils that are rich in Essential fatty acids (EFAs), Virgin Coconut Oil rich in Medium Chain Fatty Acid (MCFA) and ketogenic diet can be taken internally to boost the immune system. Walking, and sauna are also important adjuncts to boost metabolism together with an integrative anti-cancer lifestyle – anti-cancer diet, exercise, meditation, Qigong to foster an *anti-cancer terrain*. See *Anti-Cancer Action,* page 133.

Cannabis hemp oil is believed to treat various disorders by acting on the endocannabinoid system. The endocannabinoid system is a system of the body that controls many basic functions. It is also responsible for the effects of cannabis. It is made up of natural molecules known as cannabinoids and the pathways that they interact with. Together, these parts work to regulate a number of activities including mood, memory, sleep and appetite. See Rick Simpson cannabis hemp oil, Final Note, page 134

I would like to thank and acknowledge Dr. Joseph Gold, MD, of the Syracuse Cancer Research Institute, New York, for his research on cancer, cachexia and hydrazine sulfate which has given hope to thousands of patients with cancer who have chosen hydrazine sulfate therapy as an alternative unorthodox chemotherapy.

I would also like to thank and acknowledge Danny Orijuela, the inventor of Negative Ion device (electrotherapy device); Ralph Moss, the author of "The Cancer Industry: The Classic Expose on the Cancer Establishment," together with Morton Walker's "Cancer's Cause, Cancer's Cure," Dr. Schreiber's Anti Cancer, and Richard Walters, author of "Options: the Alternative Cancer Therapy Book." I would also like to thank and acknowledge the pharmacists Theodore G Tong and Stephen R. Saklad for their work on the Tyramine-rich foods to avoid when a patient is receiving monoamine oxidase inhibitor (MAOI) therapy such as Hydrazine Sulfate. With thanks also to Rick Simpson for his cannabis hemp oil.

May the contents of this book enlighten you about cancer and may you give Hydrazine Sulfate or medical cannabis a try as a viable option as an unorthodox chemotherapy, and also the recommended herbs (*substitutes for hydrazine sulfate* especially *Guyabano*) such as *Turmeric, Cessiac herbals, Pau d'arco, Chaparral, or Guyabano or **Dr. Beljanski's herbals (Rauwolfia Vomitoria, Pao Pereira, Ginkgo Biloba with RNA fragments) for detoxification and tonification.

Thank you for reading this book and bless you. God has not given a disease for which there is no remedy. The cure and cause of cancer is within you.

*"Turmeric (*Curcumin*) has been shown to exhibit antioxidant, anti-inflammatory, antiviral, antibacterial, antifungal, anti-angiogenesis and anticancer activities and thus has a potential against various malignant diseases, diabetes, allergies, arthritis, Alzheimer's disease, and other chronic illnesses," according to the study in *Advanced Experimental Medical Biology*. **Risk information**: Curcumin should not be taken with anti-coagulant medications or anti-inflammatory drugs. See "Turmeric, the Queen of All Herbs" at keystohealing.ca

**A recently published abstract confirms that the two plant extracts, *Pao Pereira* and *Rauwolfia vomitoria* inhibit cancer cell growth, even in those cells resistant to drugs used in chemotherapy. The results also show that healthy cells were not negatively affected, thus demonstrating the safety of the plant extracts prepared by the Beljanski method. (*Integrative Medicine and Health, May 2012)* See *beljanski.com* and *natural-source.com*

Most ailments especially cancer and kidney diseases are the result of an imbalance in the body's electrical Wei Qi field, usually due to a drop in supply of anions or negatively charged ions. Guolin Qigong and electromagnetic healing therapy can replenish the negative ions.

IMPORTANT NOTE to build your Qi, treat stress and disease integratively by yourself, and experience Self-realization through meditation and Qigong, the seven books in *You Hold the Keys to Healing* are a must read: Return to Oneness with Shiva, Return to Oneness with the Tao, Return to Oneness with Spirit through Pan Gu Shen Gong, Keys to Healing and Self-Mastery according to the Hathors, Meditation and Qigong Mastery, Oneness with Shiva, and The Cure & Cause of Cancer.

YOU HOLD THE KEYS TO HEALING

"Awareness and intention are powerful factors for personal transformation and healing."

Now that the seven books by Ricardo B Serrano have been published, Meditation and Qigong Mastery, Return to Oneness with the Tao, Return to Oneness with Spirit through Pan Gu Shen Gong, Keys to Healing and Self-Mastery according to the Hathors, Return to Oneness with Shiva, Oneness with Shiva, and The Cure & Cause of Cancer, the important questions are, what makes these books different from other related meditation and Qigong books? What will you learn from reading these books?

These seven books have the same goal: to offer readers how-to-techniques to manage stress in their daily lives and spiritually awaken when stress is cleared and released. These keys to your healing - are the non-sectarian how-to-techniques that have been personally practiced and developed for 30 years by the author, Ricardo B Serrano, and have been tested in clinical setting by him, his clients, and other Taoist, Buddhist and Yoga meditation and Qigong practitioners of every pantheistic - All is God - tradition for centuries for healing and personal transformation.

The first book Meditation and Qigong Mastery elaborates on the meditation and Qigong principles that masters use to activate and develop their lightbodies, also called EMF (electromagnetic fields), Wei Qi or merkaba, which is the missing mastery principle not discussed by eastern authors in their meditation and Qigong books. Omkabah heart lightbody activation and Maitreya (Shiva) Shen Gong are introduced. Quotations on inner mastery by meditation masters are included to guide the readers toward the path of inner mastery. Powerful mantras are also included to unite the meditation practitioners to the spiritual divine energy of the ancient lineage of the Siddha and Buddhist Masters. Lastly, the merkaba energy ball of light with holographic sound healing is taught for healing and spiritual awakening.

The second book Return to Oneness with the Tao elaborates on the Taoist meditation and Qigong inner alchemy techniques such as lower dantien breathing, Microcosmic Orbit Qigong, primordial wuji Qigong, meditation on twin hearts, and Tibetan Shamanic Qigong to cultivate the Three Treasures Jing, Qi and Shen. An important addition to this book is the understanding of a most important principle - awareness and intention are powerful factors for personal transformation and healing. When we are aware of what is - the emotional root cause of disease that is blocking the flow of Qi - we can intentionally release it through meditation and Qigong to effect a process of change for personal transformation and healing.

"God Consciousness is the reality of everything." - Shiva Sutra 1.1

The third book Return to Oneness with Spirit through Pan Gu Shen Gong elaborates on the use of Pan Gu Shen Gong together with the EFT Qi-healer's Method to effectively clear and release the emotional debris held in the body, cultivate the Three Treasures Jing, Qi and Shen, and strengthen one's self-awareness through an integrated combination of Toltec wisdom, Qigong, Qi-healing, emotional freedom technique therapy, ear acupuncture, and Chinese tonic herbs. We are sick because we are not aware. Awareness is the key to healing.

The goal of the fourth book Keys to Healing and Self-Mastery according to the Hathors, a supplementary book to Holographic Sound Healing taught at the Meditation and Qigong Mastery book, and the Omkabah Heart Lightbody Activation video, is to build the Ka and offer readers an effective Hathor's emotional mastery technique to manage emotional stress, the main cause of disease, in their daily lives and spiritually awaken when emotional stress is cleared, released and stabilized. Doing this practice will provide a fast, safe way to stabilize your chaotic emotions such anger or fear. Holographic Sound Healing with the Four Sacred Elements is integrated with Ka(Merkaba) Meditation to complement Holographic Lightbody activation, and build the Sahhu or immortal golden lightbody. Dr. Johanna Budwig's Diet for Cancer and Chronic Diseases and Sun gazing are included as adjunct keys to healing.

The goal of the fifth book Return to Oneness with Shiva is to offer a solution to most people whose life challenge is battling their monkey-mind (ego) which I believe is the cause of suffering and can be conquered by becoming like Hanuman whose love and devotion to his Sadguru is shown by the application of Hanuman Qigong and Hunaman ji's mantras and self-realization teachings of Kashmir Shaivism. Healing with the hologram of love merkaba energy ball of light encoded with the healing conscious mind encodements is also included. Who and what you meditate on, you become.

The important questions: "Who am I? Why was I born? What is the goal of my life? What am I supposed to accomplish here?" are hopefully answered in the sixth book Oneness with Shiva, the supplementary book to the "Return to Oneness with Shiva" with the help of my Siddha Guru Baba Muktananda's excerpts from his books and my Sadguru Nityananda's grace which are based from the Self-realization teachings of Kashmir Shaivism. Who and what you meditate on, you become. When you meditate on the Self as the Self, you become one with Shiva, the Self of all.

The final seventh book "The Cure & Cause of Cancer: An Alternative Holistic Approach to Heal Cancer," is focused on the therapeutic measures to heal cancer manifesting in the body through the Budwig diet, Cessiac herbal formulas, electrotherapy, alkaline water, coconut oil, reishi mushroom, cannabis and other tonic herbs to detox the body and boost the body's Wei Qi immune system fostering an anti-cancer terrain. Oriental medical therapies such as acupuncture, acupressure, pranic healing, meditation and Qigong are also used to balance and build the body's Qi.

In summary, the seven books Meditation and Qigong Mastery, Return to Oneness with the Tao, Return to Oneness with Spirit, and Keys to Healing and Self-Mastery according to the Hathors, Return to Oneness with Shiva, Oneness with Shiva, and The Cure & Cause of Cancer form a strong basic foundation, so to speak, of dietary and energy-based psychoneuroimmunolgy or neuroimmunomodulation strategies to effectively heal substance abuse and chronic diseases mainly caused by emotional stress, diet that is high in trans-fatty acids and low in Essential Fatty Acids, and unhealthy lifestyle. These strategies bring the physical, mental, emotional, and spiritual aspects of a person into homeostasis, and at the same time spiritually awaken a person in the process of being in the flow because the individual being is one with universal being.

The reality of this whole universe is God consciousness. It is filled with God consciousness. This world is nothing but the blissful energy of the all-pervading consciousness of God. God and the individual are one, to realize this is the essence and goal of meditation and Qigong.

Whatever the diagnosis of your disease, you do not have to expect the worst. For every problem, there are solutions. You hold the keys to healing.

The seven books: Meditation and Qigong Mastery, Return to Oneness with the Tao, Return to Oneness with Spirit through Pan Gu Shen Gong, Keys to Healing and Self-Mastery according to the Hathors, Return to Oneness with Shiva, Oneness with Shiva, and The Cure & Cause of Cancer comprise altogether my Master Pranic Healer thesis for the Integral Studies of Inner Sciences.

The *Atma (Soul) Yoga of Immortality*, founded by Acharya Ricardo B Serrano, which is about becoming a Self-realized soul by attaining oneness with the Higher Soul also uses the seven books in the curriculum of the Integral Studies of Inner Sciences.

Why should we know the origin of rivers? Our duty is to bathe in them, to wash away our impurities, and to cool the heat of our bodies. In the same way, it is our duty to understand the sages, to contemplate their teachings, and to practice the sadhana (spiritual practices) which they have shown us. It is our duty to attain our own divinity, to become happy in the bliss of reunion with the Self, and to lead our lives with great freedom and joy. Above all, our task is to complete our journey to the Self. Harboring unnecessary doubts makes a person fall from the path. Source: Oneness with Shiva by Acharya Ricardo B Serrano, R.Ac., page 49

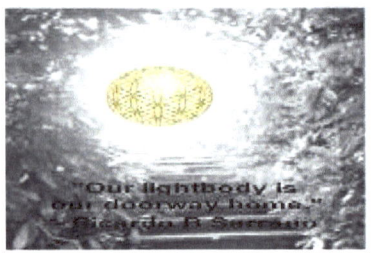

ELECTROTHERAPY

A list of patients with testimonials were cured by electro-therapy device, a machine which discharges negative ions or atoms with negative charge. Negative ions neutralize toxins in the cells and help revitalize the body.

The machine generates negative ions that are applied directly on the skin. The ions help purify the blood and take out toxins through urination, defecation, vomiting or perspiration.

The electro therapy device is also called negative ion device because it releases negative current through the skin by using conductors, which are stainless aluminum plates. It has an amplifier or booster. Simply, it is a combination of electricity which is purified, with only the negative charge retained. It has an amplifier to boost the charge, and it also uses earth so that the patient would not be electrocuted or burned.

It involves applying negative ions on the human body through electrotherapy without harming the body, to neutralize biochemical toxins, viruses, bacteria, parasites and even cancer cells.

The machine also stimulates the cells, tissues, organs and at the same time strengthens the immune system, giving it the capacity to treat never before cured diseases.

Negative ions surround the environment. An area with high concentration of these particles also has a high concentration of oxygen, an element essential for respiratory and cardiovascular systems.

Other inventions such as air conditioning units filters, television monitor screens, laundry aide, and hygienic products also use negative ions to protect people from radiation and toxins.

The device also restores balance in human health. It provides added negative ions to the cells. Once the ions fall below the normal level, people get sick. So this electro therapy device serves as self-charger.

The device can also break up embolism and formations of blood, fats and sugar in the body. The use of electro therapy device works well with support treatment program, including cleansing or alkaline diet. This is a combination of food and electro therapy.

Diseases recur and are not treated by western medicine. It is especially designed and constructed for incurable diseases. Acupuncture, herbs, Qigong are adjuncts to electrotherapy. The machine treats numerous conditions such as stroke, cancer, paralysis, arthritis, muscle pain, gout, diabetic pain and others that could not be cured by drugs.

Source: Negative Ion Therapy by Danny Orijuela, Natural doctor and inventor of electrotherapy

Photobiomodulation is a form of light therapy that utilizes non-ionizing light sources, including lasers, light emitting diodes, and/or broadband light, in the visible (400 – 700 nm) and near-infrared (700 – 1100 nm) electromagnetic spectrum. Light energy is Qi. Light therapy is a form of Qi-healing. See Intranasal Light Therapy, pages 111, 135

Intranasal light therapy with 633 nm, stimulates the mitochondria to produce more ATP, and triggers the release of nitric oxide (NO), a powerful cell signaler and activator. NO sends "blood flow signals" that relax arterial walls, dilate the blood vessels, and improve the flow of blood and oxygen everywhere in your body, boosting its ability to heal obesity, heart disease, cancer, Alzheimer's, stroke, arthritis, high blood pressure, and of course diabetes.

Intranasal light therapy devices consist of three models: **633 Red** (LED) and **655 Prime** (low-level laser) for systemic use, and **810** Infrared for brain stimulation. Acupuncture, herbs, diet, exercise, and Qigong are adjuncts to intranasal light therapy.

The amyloid plaques in the neurons of Alzheimer's brain are removed by photobiomodulation. The Default Mode Network disruptions in the areas of the brain are also targeted and normalized. Photobiomodulation by Vielight Neuro Gamma is a non-drug effective approach that not only works for Alzheimer's but also works for: anxiety, depression, insomnia, brain injury, CTE, PTSD, stroke, autism, ADHD, Parkinson's, psychosis, addictions, attain higher meditative states and athletic performance.

If I get Cancer, in a Nutshell

Truthfully, the second reason for writing this book is not only for the benefit of other people but also for myself, too.

I have told my wife that if I get cancer, God forbid, I will never be put under the care of medical doctors whose only symptomatic treatment options for cancer are chemotherapy, radiation and surgery. I have told her that I will follow the method outlined in this book when I get cancer as soon as possible to have better prognosis and results.

Killing cancer is like killing those voracious mosquitos whose numbers keep increasing despite the method in killing those pesky blood suckers. The best way is to wear proper clothing and sleep in mosquito nets to prevent them from sucking your blood's nutrients for their sustenance. In the same way, it is a much more practical common sense to starve those voracious cancer cells to use glucose by taking the anti-cachexia hydrazine sulfate or medical cannabis that inhibit gluconeogenesis and stop the wasting syndrome – cachexia, rather than poisoning them with toxic chemotherapy which are fatal not only to cancer cells but also to normal cells.

I would also use an electromagnetic healing machine that can supply negative ions since most ailments especially cancer and kidney diseases are the result of an imbalance in the body's electrical Wei Qi field, usually due to a drop in supply of anions or negatively charged ions.

The electrotherapy device is described as a multi-functional machine invented in the Philippines that can stimulate and rebuild the body's natural electric field. Safety precautions and expert guidance for its use are recommended. Intranasal light therapy can be used with the electrotherapy device. See Negative Ion Therapy, pages 103, 108, 111

And of course, I will make changes in my lifestyle and take care of myself better by eating a ketogenic diet (a high fat low-carb diet), follow the Budwig diet (cottage cheese with fresh oils rich in EFAs) and take *Virgin Coconut Oil*, take reishi mushroom, hemp oil, *Turmeric*, Green tea, Cessiac herbals, aratiles, Pau d'arco, Chaparral, Guyabano with alkaline water, and of course, avoid stress and regularly do walking Qigong (Guo Lin Qigong) and practice meditation and Qigong with emotional healing I have outlined as holistic approach described in my seven books in *You Hold the Keys to Healing*.

The aratiles fruit is known in other countries as Jamaican cherry, Panama berry, Singapore cherry, bolaina yamanaza, cacaniqua, capulín blanco, nigua, niguito, memizo, or memiso. In certain areas of the Philippines, these little red fruits are called manzanitas ("small apples"), also spelled mansanitas or manchanitas

Kerson Fruit or Muntingia calabura (aratiles) is a fast growing tree that has a cherry like fruit with multiple health benefits: Such as antibacterial, lowering blood sugar, preventing cancer, promoting cardiovascular health, lowering blood pressure, and blocking pain (gout, headaches) ... just to name a few. According to research, the leaves of the Kerson tree demonstrates great anti-cancer abilities and may be utilized more widely in the future for cancer cure – additional studies required.

I will regularly go for sauna, visit my acupuncturist friends to have acupuncture treatment, visit my pranic healer friends to have pranic healing session, and practice meditation and Qigong with my meditation and Qigong friends to replenish the negative ions in my Wei Qi field.

If things get worse, which I doubt will ever happen, at least I will be ready mentally, emotionally and spiritually to leave this physical world – what's wrong with dying anyways? and meet my loved ones in heaven, our true spiritual home. My mother used to say, God helps those who help themselves. God is within you!

How to Conquer Death Now

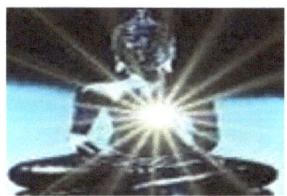

"We have to realize our identity with the Universal Consciousness. We have to merge with that Consciousness, just as a river merges with the ocean. When a being has attained this state of oneness, he has gone beyond death."

- Swami Muktananda Paramahamsa

May the following Kashmir Shaivism based excerpts from the book "Does Death Really Exist?" by Swami Muktananda Paramahamsa enlighten those people seeking answers to the ever most important question: how to conquer death - end the cycle of death and rebirth - in this lifetime. I believe that we can conquer death now by returning to oneness - uniting our individual consciousness with the universal consciousness through the practice of meditation and Qigong.

Excerpts from Does Death Really Exist? by Swami Muktananda Paramahamsa:

How can a person free himself from this wheel of death and rebirth? He can do so only by going within and through meditation discovering his own inner Self. As we meditate, we become established in the seat of the inner Self, and then we are liberated from death. In meditation, we discard our individual ego and merge with the Self. The ego is a veil which hides the Self and keep us bound to the body. The ego is nothing but our sense of limited individuality, an identification with the body and the mind, with our sex, our family, our country, our position. Although the Self is completely stainless, when it is enveloped in the three impurities (malas) the ego is born, and we become bound.

The purpose of spiritual life is to become free of these impurities, and to do that we must perform only good actions. If we perform bad actions - if we hurt ourselves or other people - then over and over again we are enveloped by these malas. As long as we are covered by them, we are mere human beings. But once we become free of them, we are nothing but Supreme Consciousness.

Within every human being is a great and divine energy called Kundalini (Shakti)... When it is awakened through the grace of the Guru, a spontaneous process begins within. Then the awakened energy moves through our system, burning all the impurities in the body. Through the meditation which takes place after Kundalini awakening, one easily comes to see the Self within the heart. The fire of that knowledge of the Self destroys the three malas, and one expands more and more. Once one has completely evolved, one knows, "I am God." Instead of having the awareness that one is the body, one very naturally becomes aware, "I am the Self." When one realizes that God dwells within as one's own inner Self, the fire of that knowledge burns all one's accumulated karma...

"Because of the three malas - anavamala (awareness of imperfection), mayiyamala (awareness of duality), and karmamala (awareness of doership) - an individual soul is born again and again. When the malas are removed through spiritual practices and the grace of a pure being, the individual soul goes beyond birth and death and is never born again.

"The truth is that it is our own ego which is death for us. When we have gone beyond the ego, death no longer exists.

"In the same way, our ego brings us again and again to our death. In order to conquer death, we have to transcend the ego, to overcome our limited individuality. We have to realize our identity with the Universal Consciousness. We have to merge with that Consciousness, just as a river merges with the ocean. When a being has attained this state of oneness, he has gone beyond death. The Gita says: "The embodied one, having gone beyond the three gunas - sattva (purity), rajas (activity), and tamas (inertia) - out of which the body is evolved, is freed from birth, death, decay, and pain and attains immortality."

"Whatever being a person thinks of at the last moment when he leaves his body, that alone does he attain." Therefore, whatever is in one's mind at the moment of death is extremely significant. For this reason we hold regular recitation of sacred texts at our Ashrams. If one memorizes good words, they keep reverberating inside. If one studies the Bhagavad Gita, the Bible, and the Upanishads, they keep coming to one's mind. One who remembers God constantly in this way will attain the state of God at the time of death. One who meditates and prays every day has no fear of death.

We forget to contemplate, "Who am I? Why was I born? What is the goal of my life? What am I supposed to accomplish here?" We forget the reason we are here, and we eat and drink and make merry. We indulge in sense pleasures, and one day we leave this body. Kabir wrote: "O friend, listen to me: through chanting God's name, great beings go across in this way. One day the body will drop away. In this world, everything that comes also goes. But the Self does not die. The inner Self is ageless and unchanging. Death cannot reach it. Therefore, live with the awareness: "The Supreme Truth lies within me; the flame of Supreme Truth is shimmering and shining inside me." That light is the Self.

May your awareness turn inward. May you live with the knowledge, "I am the Supreme Truth; pure Consciousness lies within me." Through the fire of knowledge, may death die for you. I wish this for you all.

Within this body the taintless string of beads goes round and round day and night.

It goes up and down with each breath.

Not understanding this, worldly people let their breath go to waste and walk into the jaws of death.

Without the aid of tongue or teeth every living being repeats the So'ham mantra.

Day and night, awake or sleep, it doesn't stop even for a moment.

Hamsa-So'ham, Hamsa-So'ham – it goes on and on.

The Sadguru unravels its secret and makes your mind still.

Brahmananda says: "Yogis who sit and meditate on this every morning attain the state of liberation. They are not born again."

"Finally, as you pursue this self-born yoga, as the inner Shakti unfolds, you reach the sahasrara, the topmost spiritual center in the crown of the head. This is the culmination of the spiritual journey, and here the light of the Self reveals itself. In the sahasrara there is a divine effulgence. That light has the radiance of a thousand suns. In that center, there is no pain and no pleasure. Only the bliss of consciousness exists there. In the center of that divine effulgence in the sahasrara, there is a tiny subtle blue light, which yogis call the nila bindu, the blue pearl. Watching this tender, infinitely fascinating light, you become aware of your true glory. Though smaller than a sesame seed, the blue pearl contains the entire universe. It is the light of God, the form of God within you. This is the divinity, this is the greatness that lies within a human being…Therefore, perceive that light. Only if you discover that light will you recognize who you truly are." – Muktananda

Cannabis and Strokes

According to Dr. David Allen, the leading causes of strokes are high blood pressure, atherosclerosis, a weak heart, and simply the accumulated wear and tear of age. For those who survive a stroke, symptoms include difficulty speaking or full loss of speech, memory impairments, motor (movement) issues, paralysis (paraplegia, quadriplegia), challenges in writing, and even changes in personality.

Treating Atherosclerosis

Atherosclerosis, a condition in which an artery wall thickens and smooth muscle cells appear that result in a fatty plaque — which eventually blocks arterial blood flow and can lead to a blockage — is one of the leading causes of stroke and heart diseases. Research has shown cannabinoids to be an effective treatment for atherosclerosis, helping prevent a stroke from occurring in the first place.

A study published in the journal Nature in 2005 revealed that THC, even in low quantities, when acting on the CB2 receptors found throughout the immune system, decreased the severity of a stroke.

"Oral administration of THC (1 mg kg-1 per day) resulted in significant inhibition of disease progression. This effective dose is lower than the dose usually associated with psychotropic effects of THC. Thus, THC or cannabinoids with activity at the CB2 receptor may be valuable targets for treating atherosclerosis."

Another study conducted in 2007 and published in the American Journal of Physiology revealed that the cannabinoid CBD was effective in dealing with inflammation and other symptoms of atherosclerosis. Reported the study:

"Our results suggest that CBD, which has recently been approved for the treatment of inflammation, pain, and spasticity associated with multiple sclerosis in humans, may have significant therapeutic benefits against diabetic complications and atherosclerosis."

Dr. David Allen

In those who do suffer strokes, the administration of CBD and THC prior to onset can decrease the severity of the stroke significantly. Dr. David Allen, a former heart surgeon, when referring to cannabis in the treatment of stroke and heart disease, said "No other medicine made by man can help in this manner."

Allen cites a government patent from 2003 that reveals that the administration of cannabinoids prior to the onset of a stroke can decrease its severity by about 50 percent. Said Dr. Allen:

"No other chemical decreases the size of a stroke by even two percent. So this is like a miracle that it does this."

Allen adds that it's "nearly impossible to come back from many strokes." Thus, any treatment, such as cannabinoids, that can decrease the severity of a stroke may serve to preserve life-giving cognitive and neurological functions, as well as critical motor skills. Instead of aspirin to thin the blood and decrease the chances of a blockage, Allen recommends cannabis to his patients. "Eat a bud a day, it keeps the stroke away," said Allen.

See About Medical Cannabis, page 17; How Medical Cannabis Works, page 19; Holistic Biochemistry of Cannabinoids, page 20; How and Why Garlic Works, page 61; Reishi Mushroom, page 63

Negative Ion Therapy

If you are desperately ill or hopelessly sick and modern medicine including surgery gives you little or no help, you may think you need a miracle to get back your health. This "miracle" may be provided by Qigong and a new electromagnetic healing technology that promises to correct what is wrong with your body especially cancer, kidney diseases, fatigue, high blood pressure, viral infections. Most ailments are the result of an imbalance in the body's electrical Wei Qi field, usually due to a drop in supply of anions or negatively charged ions.

Qigong aims to correct this imbalance by bombarding the body with anions or negative ions from nature until the right yin-yang balance is achieved. When this is accomplished, the human body will go back to its normal functioning self, free of any disease. See Nature generates negative ions, page 115

Another way to correct the ionic imbalance is by an electrotherapy device which is described as a multi-functional machine invented in the Philippines that can stimulate and rebuild the body's natural electric field. Safety precautions and expert guidance for its use are recommended.

The negative ions are provided by electricity from an electromagnetic healing machine that is strapped for a number of hours each day through the Laogong point (Pericardium 9) of the hands and in the feet in the Yong Quan point (Kidney 1) of the patient supplying the healing Qi into the kidneys' adrenals building the Yuan Qi. This is similar to the effect of internal and external Qigong in the body's storage of Source Qi in the lower dantian to cultivate the Three Treasures Jing, Qi and Shen for healing and enlightenment.

The electrotherapy device together with coco keto diet, exercise and lifestyle change can assist the body to heal chronic conditions such as arthritis, gout, asthma, emphysema, numbness, pneumonia, extending lifespan of cancer patients, diabetic complications, infectious diseases, patients with alzheimer's and parkinson's, kidney failure patients undergoing kidney dialysis, neuralgia, autism, heart enlargement, stroke, hepatitis, hypertension and other diseases.

Ionic detox foot bath and Far Infrared (FIR) therapy restore the body's Qi by changing the pH from acidic toward alkaline. Ionic detox helps to facilitate the alkalization process through ionization which removes "free radicals" from the body. Ionic detox is especially good for those suffering from GI disorders, skin conditions, yeast or fungal infections and cancer. FIR induces hyperthermia that elevates local body temperature which increases circulation promoting healing and detoxification. Ionic detox foot bath and FIR therapy provide the following benefits: Increases energy level; significant pain control; improves sleep and memory; cleanses kidney, liver and parasites in our body; enhances immune system; liver detoxification which cleanses overall body; normalize blood pressure and increases blood circulation; alleviates allergies; helps weight reduction; increases metabolism and reduce constipation.

Why do Qigong, Pranic Healing and Intranasal Light Therapy work?

What is reality? "What we have called matter is energy (light), whose vibration has been so lowered as to be perceptible to the senses. There is no matter." - Albert Einstein

"If you want to find the secrets of the universe, think in terms of energy, frequency and vibration." - Nikola Tesla

"The knower and the known are one. Simple people imagine that they should see God as if he stood there and they here. This is not so. (...) The eye with which I see God is the same eye with which God sees me. My eye and God's eye is one eye, and one sight, and one knowledge, and one Love." – Meister Eckhart

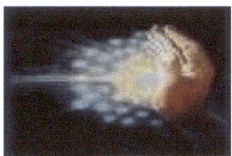

Healing Cancer with Pranic Healing

A cancerous organ or part is clairvoyantly seen as dark muddy yellow and red. There is too much yellow and red prana in the affected area, resulting in the rampant growth of cancerous cells. This condition is brought about by an overactive basic chakra, meng mein chakra, and solar plexus chakra. Although these chakras are overactivated, they are very depleted. Anger, resentment, hatred or fear activates the solar plexus area. The overactivated solar plexus chakra in turn activates the meng mein and basic chakras. This, in the long run, may manifest as cancer. It seems that negative emotions in the form of long-standing anger, resentment, hatred or fear is a major contributing cause of cancer.

1. Apply general sweeping several times. Many cancer patients, if not all, have blackish or darkish gray auras. The outer, health, and inner auras are badly affected.
2. Inhibit the overactivated but depleted solar plexus, meng mein and basic chakras. This is very important in order to correct the condition causing the rapid growth of cancer cells. Apply localized sweeping and energizing on the solar plexus chakra with green, violet and dark blue prana. Then inhbit the solar plexus chakra by willing the solar plexus chakra to become smaller (about three inches in diameter) while energizing with dark blue prana.

Apply localized sweeping and energizing thoroughly on the basic and meng mein chakras with light green prana, light whitish-violet prana, then with dark blue prana. Inhibiting the meng mein and basic chakras is done by willing these chakras to become two-and-a-half inches in diameter while energizing with dark blue prana. The solar plexus, basic and meng mein chakras usually become overactivated again after a day or two. This is why treatment has to be repeated three times a week.

3. To enhance the defense mechanism of the body, clean the bones in the arms and legs thoroughly by applying localized sweeping. Energize the sole, knee, and hip chakras with light whitish-violet prana, and visualize pranic energy going inside the bones. Energize the hand, elbow, and armpit chakras with light violet and visualize the pranic energy going inside the bones.
4. Clean, energize and activate the crown, forehead, ajna, back head, and throat chakras with light green, light blue and light violet prana. When energizing with light violet prana, will the crown, forehead, ajna, and throat chakras to become bigger (about five or six inches in diameter) and the back head chakra to about two inches in diameter. This is to activate the upper chakras in order to produce more green, blue, and violet prana, which have neutralizing effects on cancer cells.
5. Clean the front and back heart chakras thoroughly. Energize the back heart chakra with light whitish-violet prana and simultaneously will the heart chakra to become five or six inches in diameter, this will help the patient experience a sense of inner peace.
6. Apply cleansing on the affected parts. This is done by applying localized sweeping on the affected part about one to two hundred times. This will partially or completely relieve the patient of pain. Be sure to wash your hands regularly while cleansing. You must remember that the affected part is very dirty, congested, and filled with dark muddy red and yellow pranas. Energize the affected part with dark blue prana for about fifteen minutes in order to inhibit the growth of cancer cells and to localize them. Also inhibit the affected part which is overactivated. Energize the affected part with your finger with dark green prana, then with dark orange prana about five minutes each. Visualize the pranic energy coming out as laser-like and as thin as the tip of a ball point. The dark green prana, and dark orange prana have to be projected in a very concentrated form to give it sufficient potency to partially disintegrate the cancer cells. Do not use orange prana on delicate organs.

7. Repeat the treatment three times a week for five months, or for as long as necessary. The treatment should not be done too frequently because the patient might be overenergized and healing process might be slowed down.

Encourage the patient to become a vegetarian. Aside from the benefits derived from a vegetarian diet, being a vegetarian is an act of showing mercy toward the animal kingdom. Based on the law of karma, a person who shows mercy will also in turn receive mercy. This encourages faster healing of the illness. Furthermore, instruct the patient to practice *Meditation on Three Hearts* regularly to help generate more positive karma.

The following are the benefits derived by cancer patients from this form of healing: the intense pain will be gradually reduced after several treatments; the energy level of the patient will be increased and the patient will feel much stronger after several treatments. The appetite will improve; the growth of the cancer cells will be reduced if not stopped; and the cancer cells will be gradually and partially destroyed. For terminal cancer patients, pranic healing will enable them to die in peace and with dignity,

Some cancer patients cannot be healed for a number of reasons. The patient's body may have already been badly damaged by potent drugs. The cancer cells may have already spread; or the body is extremely weak and its capacity to absorb and retain pranic energy has greatly diminished. Sometimes organ(s) have been badly damaged that they are beyond repair. And last, the ailment could be of karmic origin. Because of these factors, some cancer patients will be partially or completely relieved, their health improved, and their life prolonged, but only a few will be completely cured.

Source: Pranic Healing by Grand Master Choa Kok Sui, 1990.

MEDITATION ON THREE HEARTS

1. Clean the etheric body, do physical exercise for about 5 minutes.
2. Invoke for divine blessing.

Father, I humbly invoke Thy divine blessing! For protection, guidance, help and illumination! With thanks and full faith.

3. Activate the heart chakra, together with sex chakra connected to earth, concentrate on them, and bless the entire earth with loving-kindness.

From the heart of God,

Let the entire earth be blessed with loving-kindness.

Let the entire earth be blessed with great joy, happiness and divine peace.

Let the entire earth be blessed with understanding, harmony, good will and will to do good. So be it!

From the heart of God,

Let the hearts of all sentient beings be filled with divine love and kindness.

Let the hearts of all sentient beings be filled with great joy, happiness and divine peace.

Let the hearts of all sentient beings be filled with understanding, harmony, good will and will to do good. With thanks, so be it!

4. Activate the crown chakra, concentrate on it, and bless the entire earth with loving-kindness. Then bless the earth with loving-kindness simultaneously through the crown, heart chakra and sex chakra.
5. To achieve illumination, concentrate on the point of light, on top of the head, on the Aum, and on the gap between the two Aums.
6. To release excess energy, bless the earth with light, love and peace.
7. Give thanks!
8. Massage the physical body, and do physical exercise for about five minutes.

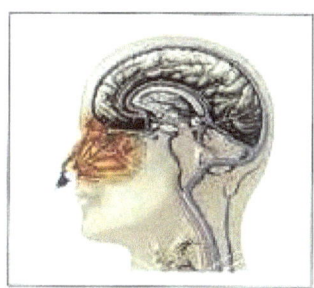

Intranasal Light Therapy by Dr. Lew Lim, ND

"Matter is Energy. Energy is Light. We are all Light Beings." - Albert Einstein

Intranasal Light Therapy involves the simple process of clipping a small red light diode to the nose to illuminate the nasal cavity. Researchers have found that this act initiates the process of healing a large number of health conditions such as high blood pressure, high cholesterol, diabetes and viral infection. How can such a simple device be so effective in healing so many diseases? In fact, the Intranasal Light Therapy device does only one thing, and it does it well. It stimulates the body to heal itself. The impact is systemic rather than directed at any particular condition. And in the process, many conditions are addressed.

Scientists who specialize in the stimulation characteristic of light (or "photobio-stimulation") know that a certain wavelength of light can trigger the creation of singlet oxygen. At low dosage, these singlet oxygen particles settle into "Redox Signalling" molecules. These signalling molecules tell the body to line up its various elements to accomplish the following healing activities: activate the immune system, release antioxidants, increase blood flow, repair damaged DNA, and even encourage the death of damaged cells.

With Intranasal Light Therapy, this effect commences with the blood passing through the nasal region and then continues to spread throughout the body via the circulatory and lymphatic systems.

The reduction-oxidation ("redox") activities continuously take place inside the body, but when inflammation occurs due to an infection, or when cellular homeostasis (equilibrium of interdependent elements) is interrupted, the body's corrective system is called into action. The redox signalling (stimulated by light therapy as explained here) helps the body to more accurately direct this restorative action. The result is accelerated healing, or the body being put on alert.

There are no major side effects with this therapy. Nor does it require the introduction of a foreign substance into the body. The healing process is completely natural in harnessing the power of the body to repair itself. Intranasal Light Therapy is low-cost, effective and convenient, which makes it a healing breakthrough. It is a natural fit with the value system of naturopathic medicine. It does no harm, respects the natural power of the body to heal, addresses the causes of illness rather than the symptoms (at the molecular level), encourages self-responsibility for health, considers the fundamental health factors, and definitely promotes prevention of diseases.

Furthermore, Intranasal Light Therapy is supported by a large body of scientific evidence illustrating its underlying mechanism and its efficacy against many diseases. In China, the Intranasal Light Therapy technology is certified by the government. Ten million of these devices have been sold over the past few years, and they are used in many Chinese hospitals. North America deserves to hear about this. **See Intranasal Light Therapy, page 135**

To enter higher states of consciousness, I use intranasal light therapy with kundalini meditation and Qigong. - Ricardo B Serrano, R.Ac.

Photobiomodulation is a natural way to heal diseases and enhance brain function.

"I take Chinese herbs and practice acupressure, Qigong with intranasal light therapy, and don't take prescription drugs because of its toxic side-effects and addictive nature. So, traditional Chinese medicine works for me." – Ricardo B Serrano, R.Ac.

Get Well Verse (for Cancer patients)

When in cancer, not be sad, To raise spirit is superior.

- Surgical opportunities not let missed, Chemo and Radio should be appropriate.
- Use herbs to support normality and rid the anomaly,
- When in grave sickness, don't fumble for help.
- Walking Qi Gong should be practiced, Hope still come from ill.
- Walking Qi Gong should be practiced, The whole family will rejoice in recovery.
- When in cancer, not be sad, To raise spirit is superior.
- Prevent cold, stop smoking and alcohol, Pay attention to dieting and self-care.
- Orderly routine is a blessing, An emotional setback is life's enemy.
- Walking Qi Gong should be practiced, Hope still come from ill.
- Walking Qi Gong should be practiced, The whole family will rejoice in recovery.

Oxidative stress, DNA, Telomeres, Endocannabinoid Deficiency and Guolin New Qigong

Telomeres are repeating DNA sequences located at the ends of chromosomes. With each cell division the telomeres become shorter. When the telomeres become too short, the cells stop dividing and cell death ensues. Telomeric length — shortening — is thus associated with senescence and the aging process as well as with cellular and whole-body mortality.

Oxidative stress — in the form of reactive oxygen species (ROS) — is well known to have deleterious consequences on telomeric length and therefore tissue function. Chronic oxidative stress, for example, compromises telomeric integrity and enhances the onset of senescence in human endothelial cells; this same factor accelerates telomeric loss and contributes to senescence in both human cellular and in whole-body systems.

In 2004, however, Dr. Ethan Russo proposed the idea of clinical endocannabinoid deficiency (CECD) in a study published in Neuro endocrinology letters. He suggested that deficient cannabinoid levels may be the underlying cause of numerous conditions alleviated by cannabis. Symptoms of CECD are pain, inflammation, digestive issues and anxiety and/or depression. A lifestyle of unhealthy diet, infrequent exercise, poor sleep, and lack of stress management contributes to endocannabinoid deficiency. Holistic treatment success is often attributed to activation and balancing of the body's cannabinoid receptors through cannabis, acupuncture and Qigong. See Medical Qigong, page 113

Guolin New Qigong with healthy lifestyle, diet and herbs lengthen the telomeres, builds the endocannabinoid system and thus lengthen the lives of cancer survivors and also prevent cancer and other chronic diseases.

- From the Guo Lin Qi Gong Club, China, Translated by YuanPu Zheng
- For more info on herbs, see Herbs for Cancer, page 89 and Reishi Mushroom, page 63
- For more info on Walking Qigong, see Introduction to Guo Lin Qigong, page 120
- For more info on diet, see Coconut Ketogenic Diet, page 121 with alkaline water

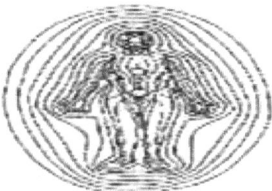

Wei Qi Field in Medical Qigong

"This field of Qi protects the body from the invasion of external pathogens and communicates with, as well as interacts with, the surrounding universal and environmental energy fields." – Chinese Medical Qigong Therapy

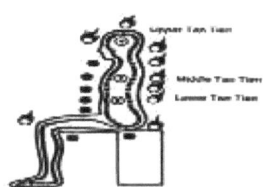

The Microcosmic Orbit is the key to balancing energies in the body to prevent kundalini syndromes, and the basic foundation for other advanced meditation practices.

I believe that Qigong also works with the body's endocannabinoid system, as does acupuncture and cannabis, since the eight extraordinary meridians are activated in the practice of Qigong manifested as a blissful high and relaxation sensation that has anti-aging health benefits to various chronic diseases.

Research is confirming that acupuncture works with the endocannabinoid system, as does Cannabis. It is not a stretch to think that if you are treating pain/inflammation with Cannabis, adding acupuncture might ease pain.

Cannabis is a non-toxic herbal medicine without side-effects and is the best alternative to prescription drugs for alleviating pain, inflammation, anxiety, depression, etc.

Cannabis has a long history in TCM. Cannabis is one of the 50 "fundamental" herbs of TCM, and is prescribed to treat diverse symptoms. Cannabis, called má, means "hemp; Cannabis; numbness" in Chinese, and was used by the Emperor Shen Nung, who was a pharmacologist. See page 134, cannabis hemp oil is used for cancer and other diseases such as high blood pressure, diabetes, asthma, depression, insomnia, inflammation, MS, addictions, etc.

Research has focused on endocannabinoid physiology. Endocannabinoids are compounds made within the body that are analogous to cannabinoids, or the plant compounds THC and CBD. At least five endocannabinoids, including anandamide, palmitoylethanolamide and 2-arachidonglycerol, have been found. Sixty-plus cannabinoids in the Cannabis plant also have potential action here. The most researched cannabinoid receptors are the cannabinoid CB1 and CB2 receptors. Significant crosstalk occurs between endogenous opiates and the endocannabinoids. These chemical signals and receptor bindings, and the TRPV1, might be how cannabinoid binding increases opiate output and vice versa.

Acupuncture influences the opioid and cannabinoid system by releasing endogenous receptor ligands. Again, the studies from the 1970's showed increased opiate production. A 2009 study that used electro-acupuncture for pain relief of inflamed skin tissue found a statistically relevant increase in anandamide (endocannabinoid) levels in the treated skin.

European researchers concluded in 2011 that "Our results suggest that electro-acupuncture reduces inflammatory pain and pro-inflammatory cytokines in inflamed skin tissues through activation of CB2 receptors." Cytokines are known as intracellular messengers, or the way cells communicate with one another. With electro-acupuncture, we get the release of endogenous opioids, increased endocannabinoids and increased activation of the cannabinoid receptors.

There are many names for the invisible auric field that surrounds the physical body in various mystical traditions such as torus, Lightbody, Electromagnetic Field (EMF), energy bubble, Merkaba or aura. The auric field is called Wei Qi Field in Medical Qigong under discussion.

According to Chinese Medical Qigong Therapy, "Qigong is a powerful system of healing and energy medicine from China. Qi means "Life-force energy" and gong means "skill," so Qigong (pronounced Chigong) is the skillful practice of gathering, circulating, and applying life-force energy. It uses breathing techniques, gentle movement, and meditation to cleanse, strengthen, and circulate the life energy or Qi and leads to better health and vitality and a tranquil state of mind. The primary goal is to purge toxic emotions from within the body's tissues, eliminate energetic stagnations, as well as strengthen and balance the internal organs and energetic fields.

All living bodies generate an external field of energy called Wei Qi (pronounced "whey chee"), which translates as "protective energy." The definition of Wei Qi in Medical Qigong is slightly different than that of Traditional Chinese Medicine (TCM). In classical TCM texts, the Wei Qi field is seen to be limited to the surface of the body, circulating within the tendon and muscle tissues. In Medical Qigong, however, the Wei Qi field also includes the three external layers of the body's auric and subtle energy fields. This energy originates from each of the internal organs and radiates through the external tissues. There the Wei Qi forms an energy field that radiates from the entire physical body. This field of Qi protects the body from the invasion of external pathogens and communicates with, as well as interacts with, the surrounding universal and environmental energy fields.

Both internal and external pathogenic factors affect the structural formation of the Wei Qi. The internal factors include suppressed emotional influences (such as anger and grief from emotional traumas). The external factors include environmental influences when they are too severe or chronic, such as Cold, Damp, Heat or Wind, etc. Physical traumas also affect the Wei Qi field.

Any negative interchange affects the Wei Qi by literally creating holes within the matrix of the individual's external energetic fields. When left unattended, these holes leave the body vulnerable to penetration, and disease begins to take root in the body. Strong emotions, in the form of toxic energy, become trapped within the body's tissues when we hold back or do not integrate our feelings. These unprocessed emotions block the natural flow of Qi, thus creating stagnant pools of toxic energy within the body.

The body has an energy field that is composed of energetic lines called meridians and channels. Energetic blockages in these channels cause imbalances in the energy field, which can lead to dis-ease. A free flow of energy is needed in the body and energy system for good health and well-being.

Medical Qigong consists of specific techniques that uses the knowledge of the body's internal and external energy fields to purge, tonify, and balance these energies. Medical Qigong therapy offers patients a safe and effective way to rid themselves of toxic pathogens and years of painful emotions that otherwise, can cause mental and physical illness. This therapy combines breathing techniques with movement, creative visualization, and spiritual intent to improve health, personal power, and control over one's own life." Internal Qigong forms (build Qi) recommended are: Pan Gu Shen Gong, Primordial Wuji Qigong, Maitreya (Shiva) Shen Gong, and Sheng Zhen Gong with Pranic Healing (Qi-healing), Eight Extraordinary Meridians Qigong, Torus Qigong with Greatest Name Chant (Gathering Qi) and Guo Lin Qigong (see page 120).

Nature generates negative ions

Why do we feel so good walking or practicing Qigong in the woods, on a beach or near a river, breathing fresh air in the mountains, or just breathing fresh air after rain or storm? Simple … We feel like that due to benign properties of negative ions abundant in these environments:

• Increase the flow of oxygen to the brain resulting in higher alertness, decreased drowsiness, and more mental energy.

• Help recovery from physical exhaustion and fatigue – achieved by increasing oxygen levels in the blood and stabilize brain function – effect – relaxation and calmness.

• Aid in blood purification by increasing the levels of calcium and sodium (healthy salt intake) in the blood stream, negative ions help restore a healthy (slightly alkaline) pH balance to the blood.

• Increase metabolism by stimulating exchange of electronic substances in cells.

• Strengthen immune system – high levels of negative ions promote production of globulin (proteins that are found extensively in blood plasma) in the blood, resulting in stronger resistance to illness.

Negative ions balance autonomic nervous system by balancing the opposing sympathetic and parasympathetic branches of the autonomic nervous system. Promote better digestion – by counteracting over-arousal of the sympathetic nervous system, negative ions help ease tension in the stomach and intestines, promoting the production of digestive enzymes and enhancing digestion. Promote cell rejuvenation by revitalizing cell metabolism, negative ions enhance vitality of muscle tissue and strengthening internal organs.

Benefits of Sheng Zhen Qigong Practice

The sacred truth - Sheng Zhen or unconditional love - can only be known by experience, not by thoughts or beliefs. Oneness or Qigong state characterized as a harmony between heaven, earth and man is experienced as a final outcome when the unhealthy Qi is completely dispelled with a Yin and Yang balance and when the Jing and Qi are plentiful in the body, and the Shen or Spirit within one's own heart opens that naturally radiate unconditional love reconnecting one's heart to the unconditional love of the universe.

According to Master Li Jun Feng's article Essence of Life, "Everyone now needs qigong. To explain what qigong is: Qi is the essence of life. It is the origin of life. With qi, everything grows. Without qi, everything dies. We believe that life comes from qi. The quality of qi affects our life. Through the practice of Real Qigong, it is good for both physical and emotional health. It stimulates the qi to flow, improving the qi exchange between the individual and nature. Through this qi flow, unhealthy qi is replaced with pure qi. When qi flows smoothly, it generates more energy in the body. Blood circulation becomes better. We believe that qi is the commander of blood - qi leads the blood to flow. When the blood flows smoothly, there is less stagnation, and the body becomes healthier.

Qigong is good for emotional health because, with the movements and understanding of the philosophy of the Real Qigong, like Sheng Zhen Wuji Yuan Gong, people understand the meaning of life better. This can remove worries and stress from their minds and bodies. Qigong changes your life to become a happy and healthy life.

Happiness and health are the essence of life. On a higher level, the main purpose of life is to learn what unconditional love is - to give more love to the world. Life comes from qi. Qi comes from the power of love. Qi and love are never separate. Each person can affect the environment, and the environment can affect the person. Each individual can positively affect the universe as a whole by sending unconditional love everywhere and to all beings. We hope unconditional love goes everywhere and to everyone. In our world, full of love, this world will become like paradise."

Glossary of Sheng Zhen Wuji Yuan Gong Terms: Baihui – the acupuncture point located at the top of the head, the center of the crown. Dantian – the storage place of Qi in the body, about two inches below the navel. Five gateways – the entry points of Qi through the palms of the hands (laogong), the soles of the feet (yongquan), and the crown of the head (baihui). Niwuan – the point located in the center of the head at the intersection between the center of the eyebrows (yintang) and the top of the head (baihui). Yintang – acupoint located at the center of the eyebrows. Zhongmai – the primordial channel in the center of the body which connects the dantian to the niwuan – the dantian being earth and the niwuan being heaven.

Anti-Aging Benefits of Qigong

"This review deals with a small fraction of the large collection of clinical research on medical applications of qigong. The information presented is intended to illustrate the potential of qigong exercise for restoring normal body functions in people with chronic conditions, many of which accelerate the aging process. The main conclusion from many studies is that qigong exercise helps the body to heal itself. In this sense, qigong is a natural anti-aging medicine. Two studies indicate that qigong exercise is superior to some physical exercises.

Qigong can complement Western medicine in many ways to provide better healthcare. For example, qigong has special value for treating chronic conditions and as a preventive medicine, whereas Western medicine has special value for treating acute conditions. There are many medical applications of qigong that can complement Western medicine to improve health care. Some examples include chronic problems such as hypertension, cardiovascular disease, aging, asthma, allergies, neuromuscular problems, and cancer. These areas of public health deserve consideration by the Western medical establishment." - Kenneth M. Sancier, PhD

See Anti-Aging Benefits of Qigong by Kenneth M Sancier, PhD of Qigong Institute at
http://qigongmastery.ca/index2.html

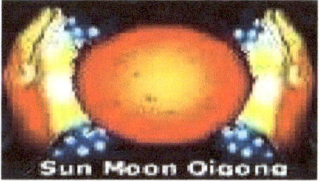

Testimonial: Pan Gu Shen Gong gives me a second chance for life

Tan Caixia, Yunan, Guangdong, China

On July 16, 2004, while traveling to Guangzhou with my husband, I suddenly felt a painful sensation throughout my bones during the trip. So when we arrived, I went to the emergency services at the Guangzhou First People's Hospital. The doctor first prescribed some painkillers, and then asked me to stay at the hospital for a further examination. After a CAT scan and a lung scan using isotopes, I was diagnosed with "mid-late lung cancer." The doctor told my husband, "You should buy more tonics for her health rather than take a surgery, for it is in vain." The nurse in charge held my hands with a message of hopeless and sympathy, saying, "Take something better when you are back home."

Back from Guangzhou, I headed to our local hospital for an injection, and took medication. Even I found a senior traditional Chinese medical doctor in Zhaoqing City to prescribe Traditional Chinese Medicine (TCM). I continually took the medicine for nearly three months, but did not become any better. My face was pale, I felt neither well-being nor power in my entire body, at the same time I became weaker gradually. At night, it was too painful to turn my body from side to side, there was just great suffering. Mostly, I had to get up to have anodyne in the mid-night so that I could sleep for a while. Every day, I relied on five to six pills of painkiller to live, but it was only a palliative. One morning, I discovered two-egg size bumps had grown both on my sternum and my right shoulder bone. It was painful when I touched them. So I began to complain to God, "Why do you treat me like this? It's too much suffering to live, better that I die rather than live!" I had to cry at home every day.

One day, my mother visited me. Seeing me in such agony, she introduced her colleague Aunt Pan to me. She said that she had practiced a miraculous qigong Pan Gu Shen gong (PGSG) for two years and gained beneficial effects, and asked if I wished to learn. I agreed that I would give it a try. After I began practicing Pan Gu Shen gong moving form, Aunt Pan and Huang helped me heal further with energy administered with the healing form. When they asked me how I felt, I could honestly answer that I felt really comfortable after healing session.

When I initially began the practice, the principle phenomenon was tears, much expectoration, fever, and sweat. However, I began to feel energetic and with power, a good appetite and less bone ache all over my body. It was better than the ease of the pain from taking the anodyne. Therefore, I gradually had to take less anodyne. After practicing only one month, I stopped all the TCM and painkillers. Later on, I learned the Non-Moving Form, and as my health was better and better, I practiced more diligently.

However, during a certain period, I was uncomfortable, cold and hot sensations brought me suffering. Especially when feeling cold, I had to cover myself with several bed quilts, but still was shaking non-stop. At that time, I thought of Huang telling me, "Never give up, no matter how painful the experience when you are practicing. Because it is normal, no need to be afraid of the experience, if you fear it, you get into a trap. You must face all the current challenges bravely, while reading more books, learn to conduct yourself as Master Ou teaches us, 'Take kindness and benevolence as basis, take frankness and friendliness to heart; speak with reason, treat with courtesy, act with emotion, accomplish result'." My heart calmed down slowly, and I continually persisted in practicing. Gradually, the cold and hot sensations disappeared.

On another day, I suddenly vomited non-stop after having a meal. I didn't know the reason, so I took the antiemetic medication. It was better hours later, and then I continually practiced. Nevertheless, the moment I recited the maxims, I started to vomit again. The situation lasted for the next ten days. I spewed such that I was not able to breathe through, all the bubbling mucus. But I felt well after that, and had a good appetite, quite different from previous experiences after vomiting, like car sickness or eating bad food. I wondered why. Then I encouraged myself to endure the suffering, and persisted in practicing with double the efforts so that I would succeed in getting through the day. It is normal to see the phenomenon that the energy from PGSG helps to exclude out the harmful elements inside the body. That's why I had vomited for days and coughed out more expectoration. I decided to stop all the medicine, and practiced wholeheartedly.

Time really flies, and I realized one day, that half a year had passed by. Through practicing PGSG regularly, reading, and conducting myself better and helping others, great changes had happened to me. The pale complexion turned to healthy red, I gained weight and add power and well-being; the bone pain gradually disappeared. I really got better! Before, I was taken care of by others, but now I could look after myself, while engaging in my family's life, actively cooking and washing. When I was out, my relatives and friends were surprised with my great changes, they couldn't imagine how I recovered so faster and was so much better from such a serious disease. In July 2006, my husband accompanied me to Guangzhou for a re-examination. The doctor and the nurse were astonished when they saw me. The nurse in charge said to me, "Wow, how fat you are?" (In Cantonese, fat is adding weight. --- by Editor) The director, who we knew in the hospital, carried the diagnosed normal lung CT and said: "How miraculous! You have such good luck as you have survived! What medicine did you take that allowed you to recover so fast?" I told him, I no longer take medicine. I just practice PGSG and that has brought me a new life. It is Pan Gu Shen gong that created this miracle!

At the beginning of practice, my husband was skeptical and wondered, "The current medicines are so efficient, but still do not cure lots of diseases. Can PGSG heal all kinds of sicknesses with such simple movements?" I disagreed with him, because many PGSG students have recovered their health through these exercises. Why not me? Later, I started to practice very diligently, more than ten or twenty times a day, even practicing until I was sleepy and ready to go to bed. Except for eating and sleeping, I spent all the time practicing the PanGu Shengong forms, reading the books of Master Ou, and taking part in team practice and exchanging ideas with other students.

Through my successful example, I have introduced my father, friends, and colleagues to learn PGSG. I hope more of those in pain can master this effective way to relieve their sufferings, and be healthy and happy. I like reading the books of Master Ou very much, for instance, The Path of Life; Farewell, my Soul; Flowers of Kindness and Beauty; and The Journey of the Heart and Soul. Sometimes, I read for students who are illiterate.

Through studying, I've learned more philosophy on how to be a healthy and happy person. Before, I was easy to lose my temper, particularly when suffering from sickness. My family were tolerant and understanding me. Now, I know that I should try my best to be a more loving person according to the maxims of PGSG, learn to be concerned about the people around me, and improve my bad temper. Seeing changes with my health and character, my husband supports me with enthusiasm instead of the previous doubt, and usually introduces others to learn PGSG.

Now I lead a good life. It is PanGu Shengong that gave me a second chance for life, enabling me to create a miracle. I feel very happy and grateful for it, and I will cherish such a not-easily-won new life. Therefore, I am determined that no matter what kinds of health adjustments might happen in the future, I should not be afraid of pains or challenges but keep practicing PGSG for several hours daily, trying to help myself, my family, and people in need. Let me live a colorful life!

Here, let me sincerely thank the deep love from PanGu Shengong and Master Ou!

Wishing all PGSG students a healthy and happy life! **Source: Pan Gu Shen Gong Newsletter**

Another Qigong for healing cancer is Guo Lin qigong that is a Kidney protection Qigong that helps to heal cancer, kidney diseases, diabetes, lung diseases, infertility, hydronephrosis, and cardiovascular diseases.

Introduction to Guo Lin Qigong by Master Sun Yun Cai (http://www.guolinqigongto.ca/)

Guo Lin Qigong, a heritage of the Chinese ancient qigong, was created by Master Guo Lin, a famous Chinese artist, based on her experiences while fighting cancer. She adopted the essence of ancient qigong and traditional Chinese medical theory about meridians (jingluo), qi (a homonym of "air" or "breath", refers to a kind of energy substance within the body) and blood. It has been practiced by thousands of people proving its benefits during recovery from cancer and in prevention of cancers, enhancing the immune system and achieving longevity. It is easy to learn and has no side effect.

Practicing Guo Lin Qigong can regulate the body and mind, and boost immune system against diseases by adjusting the body's endocrine to the best situation and enhancing the microcirculation if the practitioners practice with natural relaxation and tranquillization. Guo Lin Qigong is an oxygen absorbing exercise. It is believed that cancer cells thrive in low-oxygen environment, and high pressure oxygen can suppress or kill cancer cells and even get rid of liver cancer lumps. But inhaling too much high pressure oxygen will harm the body, so it cannot be used to treat cancer patients. Practicing Guo Lin Qigong can help creating an oxygen-rich condition in which cancer cells cannot survive. No other physical exercise or qigong can beat Guo Lin Qigong in this respect. For more info, visit (http://guolinqigong.net)

Body's internal yin and yang can be balanced, blockages of the meridians can be cleared, the flow of qi and blood can be stimulated, and body cells' electrical potential difference can be adjusted by practicing GuoLin Qigong, thus suppressing cancer cells and stimulating normal cells. Practitioners' brain activities are also better organized, thus improving vitality. So practicing Guo Lin Qigong consistently can improve our health and achieve longevity. (Read book Guo Lin Qigong – *Art of Qigong* by Zhao Jifeng)

Thousands and thousands of people are practicing Guo Lin Qigong all over the world. Among them are cancer patients, chronic disease patients and healthy persons. The Chinese Cancer Hospital of Chinese Science and Academy Institute, the Beijing Cancer Hospital, the Hong Kong Anti-Cancer Society and several hospitals in Hong Kong are using Guo Lin Qigong as one of key treatments for cancer patients during their recovery. By walking with the hands and feet moving in proper gestures, and co-ordinating with rhythmic breathing (inhaling twice and exhaling once), practitioners absorb a large quantity of oxygen so that their meridians can be regulated, flow of qi and blood can be stimulated, and their body and mind can be nourished by the nature. Thousands of practitioners suffering from medium or late stage of cancers, or chronic diseases have been cured by consistently practicing Guo Lin Qigong.

Foundation of Guo Lin Qigong (http://healthyfoundations.com/guolin/guolin_video.html)

Wheatgrass Therapy Diet: Ann Wigmore holds that the lack of enzymes is a major contributing factor in the development of leukemia and other diseases. Some of the enzymes found abundantly in raw foods diet (wheatgrass therapy diet) are cytochrome oxidase, an antioxidant required for proper cell respiration; lipase, a fat-splitting enzyme; protease, a protein digestant; amylase, which facilitates the digestion of starch; transhydrogenase, an enzyme that aids in keeping the muscle tissues of the heart toned; pepsin, which helps in digesting protein and transforming it into amino acids used for energy and self-healing; and superoxide dismutase (SOD). Richly concentrated in cereal grasses, SOD has received a lot of attention for its role in slowing cellular aging and lessening the effects of radiation. Qigong also increases SOD according to Kenneth M Sancier, PhD.

Ketogenic Diet

Many cancer patients have reportedly overcome the disease by adopting a ketogenic diet, which calls for eliminating carbohydrates, replacing them with healthy fats and protein.

Animal studies have shown that mice fed a carb-free diet survived highly aggressive metastatic cancer even better than those treated with chemotherapy.

Your normal cells have the metabolic flexibility to adapt from using glucose to using ketone bodies. Cancer cells lack this metabolic flexibility, so when you eliminate carbs, which turn into sugar, you effectively starve the cancer. Eating fat is NOT bad for your heart. Particularly, beneficial fats include virgin coconut oil, flaxseed oil, butter, organic pastured eggs, avocado, and raw nuts. Most people need as much as 50-70 percent healthful fat in their diet to optimize health.

Metabolic Therapy/Ketogenic Diet Being Investigated as Cancer Treatment

CBN News recently published an article on the ketogenic diet. Clearly, many people are realizing that what we have been doing in terms of fighting cancer is simply not working, and we cannot afford to continue in the same way. Prevention must be addressed if we ever want to turn the tide on the growing incidence of cancer across all age groups. But even more astounding, in terms of treatment, is that cancer may respond to diet alone.

"Dr. Fred Hatfield is an impressive guy: a power-lifting champion, author of dozens of books, a millionaire businessman with a beautiful wife. But he'll tell you his greatest accomplishment is killing his cancer just in the nick of time," CBN News writes. "The doctors gave me three months to live because of widespread metastatic cancer in my skeletal structure," he recalled. "Three months; three different doctors told me that same thing."

Dr. Hatfield was preparing to die when he heard of metabolic therapy, also known as the ketogenic diet. He had nothing to lose so he gave it a try, and... it worked. The cancer disappeared completely, and he'd been cancer-free for over a year.

Source: Ketogenic Diet May Be the Key to Cancer Recovery by Dr. Mercola

Adding 2 tbsp. Virgin Coconut Oil (VCO) consumption 3 to 4 X a day with the Ketogenic Diet – low carbs, high fat diet – called Coconut Ketogenic Diet is not only excellent for cancer recovery but has other health benefits as functional food explained on Virgin Coconut Oil, page 82

Avoidance of refined carbohydrates such as sugar, fructose, pop drinks is a must in this diet. Cooking with coconut oil instead of hydrogenated oils is also used in this low carb high fat diet.

Source: Coconut Ketogenic Diet by Dr. Bruce Fife, 2014 and http://www.cocoketodiet.com

Functional Medicine, Cancer, Hydrazine Sulfate and Cannabis

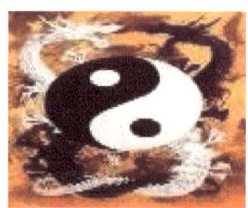

Many people who have cancer should also consider using Hydrazine Sulfate or medical cannabis even when they are using functional medicine therapies such as herbs, electrotherapy, ionic detox foot bath and FIR therapy, sauna, acupuncture, coconut ketogenic diet, meditation and Qigong. It has been said that "No reasonable hunter goes after his prey with only one bullet in his gun." And neither should a person who has cancer. Hydrazine Sulfate or medical cannabis is a powerful tool that can be effectively used for treating cancer.

Many people think that Hydrazine Sulfate or cannabis is only to be used in late stage cancer to stop a person from wasting away from cancer. This wasting away is known as cachexia. It doesn't matter if a person has cachexia or not, the cancer still responds the same way. Hydrazine sulfate or cannabis stops the cancer cell's ability to use glucose (sugar) so it helps no matter when you start using it. A person should not wait until they have the symptoms of cachexia. The longer a person waits the less likely they will recover.

Dr. Gold followed people who started using it immediately after they found out they had cancer, not waiting for the symptoms of cachexia, and these people had a 43% full recovery rate. Compare a 43% success rate to Radiation and chemotherapy's success rate of 1% to 7%.

Some people do not like the idea of using Hydrazine Sulfate because it is a chemical and yet they have no concerns about using drugs like Ibuprofen and Acetaminophen or Tylenol. When used properly all of these drugs work very well. One thing to consider is the fact that Hydrazine Sulfate or medical cannabis is hundreds of times less toxic than chemotherapy. The fact that both cannabis or hydrazine sulfate does not destroy the tissue of the body like chemotherapy or radiation makes it significantly better without any of the side effects that come from radiation and chemotherapy.

Dr. Gold discovered how well Hydrazine Sulfate worked many years ago. It has gone through phase 3 testing by the FDA but no one will finish the phase 4 testing because Hydrazine sulfate is not patentable. There have been many clinical tests done which have proven how well Hydrazine Sulfate works but still the medical profession will not fully embrace it because there is no profit in it for them. If they embraced Hydrazine Sulfate, chemotherapy and radiation would rarely be used. The lost profits from these two treatments would cause the loss of billions of dollars to doctors and hospitals.

"Functional Medicine is a true combination of Chinese Medicine, Western Medicine and scientific research. It combines the philosophy of balance and how to restore function from Chinese Medicine and the knowledge of biochemistry and physiology of Western Medicine with the latest scientific research about how our genetics, environment and lifestyle all interact with each other. Functional medicine focuses assessment and intervention at the root levels of metabolic imbalance and is an evolution in the practice of medicine that addresses the healthcare needs of the 21st century by focusing on prevention and uncovering the underlying causes of serious chronic disease. Instead of just suppressing symptoms, it deals with the root causes of disease and is less concerned with making a diagnosis and more concerned with the underlying imbalances, which are the mechanisms of the disease process.

As opposed to Western Medicine, Functional medicine treats the patient and not the disease. In addition, it provides a framework for the practice of medicine that uses all the tools of healing, both conventional and alternative, to address the whole person rather than an isolated set of symptoms. I have studied Acupuncture and Chinese Medicine which taught me to see the body from a holistic perspective. Now Functional Medicine gives me a framework to combine this with a Western understanding of the body." – Dr. Frank Lipman

Benefits of Fu Zhen Therapy and Qigong Studies of Fu Zhen herbal therapy in the United States and Canada have demonstrated its value in treating a wide range of immuno-compromised conditions, including cancer, leukemia, AIDS and ARC, and chronic Epstein-Barr virus. Fu Zhen herbs (astragalus, ligustrum, ginseng, codonopsis, atractylodes, and ganoderma) strengthen the body's nonspecific immunity and increase the function of T-cells. Kelp, turmeric (*curcumin*) and pokeroot are among the herbs known to dissolve tumors in Chinese and Ayurvedic herbal therapy.

Nobel Prize-winner Otto Warburg found that oxygen deficiency is typical of cancer cells and that when the body is rich in oxygen, cancer cells die. Practicing Qigong exercises has a positive effect on certain enzymes that play key roles in the body's maintenance of health and in *phosphorylation*, a basic biochemical process that supplies the energy for cell work. *Phosphorylation* is central to oxygen provision for all of the body's cells and is vitally important to immune response.

Exercise can mobilize the body's natural killer cells, which seek out and destroy cancer cells and cells infected by viruses. An increased oxygen uptake from the blood can also neutralize free radicals. The slow, deep breathing and moderate body motion of Qigong (or yoga) can cause the newly available oxygen to bind with free radicals, rendering them harmless. Research in China indicates that after a Qigong practice lasting about 40 minutes, the body's internal blood volume increases by 30 %, which greatly improves the supply of oxygen available to the cells.

Through intensive practice of Qigong, "a whole set of beneficial psychological and spiritual conditions emerge," observes Paul Dong in his book *Chi Gong; the Ancient Chinese Way to Health*. Besides promoting emotional well-being, Qigong exercises build patient's confidence and steel their will to defeat cancer. Dong, who has practiced Qigong since 1980, notes that positive attitude plays a role in curing disease. He likens Qigong's apparent immune-boosting effects to Western mind-body healing approaches such as the new field of *psychoneuroimmunology*.

Besides internal Qigong forms, the manipulation of energy flow within one's own body, there is also *external Qigong*, the reputed ability to project one's internal Qi toward another body. In external Qigong therapy, widely accepted in China for the treatment of many disorders, no physical contact is required. The advanced Qigong expert simply projects his or her Qi energy through the fingers or palm toward the patient, thereby purportedly killing cancer cells. External Qigong practitioners in China claim that through this technique, they can destroy bacteria and transmit health-promoting energies. They believe they have proven the existence of Qi as a physical reality evident in psychokinetic powers, clairvoyance, and healing effects. To skeptics, these assertions spring from self-deception and heightened suggestibility.

Paul Dong tells of a Japanese cancer victim, with a tumor the size of an egg deeply imbedded in his nasal cavity, who made a trip to a Beijing hospital to undergo external Qi therapy. After twelve days of treatment, the man's tumor had shrunk and his pain had considerably eased. Dr. Feng Li-da, professor of immunology at Beijing College of Traditional Chinese Medicine, has done many experiments on external Qi transmission and claims that a Qigong expert can destroy uterine cancer cells, gastric cancer cells, flu virus, and colon and dysentery bacilli with varying degrees of success. In *the Scientific Basis of Qigong*, professor Xie Huan-zhang of Beijing Industrial College states that Qi effects detected with scientific instruments include magnetic fields, infrared radiation, infrasound, and ion streams of visible light and superfaint luminescence.

Dong stresses that external Qigong Qi treatment should only be considered a temporary measure. But he also suggests that if a patient is too weak or otherwise unable to practice internal Qigong regularly, external Qi should be tried. Combinations of internal and external Qi treatment can also be attempted. Since 1979, "the Chinese have cured hundreds of cancer victims through Qigong," and many thousands have used this practice to prolong their lives, reports Paul Dong, an author and Qigong practitioner/teacher based in Oakland, California.

Source: N D Joshi, Wang Chong-xing, Roger Jahnke, and Paul Dong

Overheating Therapy

"Give me a chance to create fever and I will cure any disease." - Parmenides

Fever is one of the body's own defensive and healing forces, created and sustained for the deliberate purpose of restoring health. The high temperature speeds up metabolism, inhibits the growth of the invading virus or bacteria, and literally burns the enemy with heat. Fever is an effective protective and healing measure not only against colds and simple infections, but against such serious diseases as polio and cancer. In biological clinics, overheating therapies or artificially induced fever are used effectively in the treatment of acute infectious diseases, arthritis and rheumatic diseases, skin disorders, insomnia, muscular pain and cancer, to name a few conditions.

SAUNA

A sauna, or Finnish steam bath, is another excellent way to benefit from overheating therapy. In addition to an artificially induced fever, which a prolonged steam bath always accomplishes, the sauna bath is specifically conducive to profuse therapeutic sweating.

The skin is our largest eliminative organ - "the third kidney." It is generally considered that the skin should eliminate 30 percent of the body wastes by way of perspiration. Due to lack of physical work and overly sedentary life, the skin of most people today has degenerated as an eliminative organ, since it is hardly ever subjected to sweating. If health is to be restored, it is of vital importance that the eliminative activity of the skin is revitalized. Taking sauna or steam baths regularly, once or twice a week, will help to restore and revitalize the cleansing activity of the skin.

The therapeutic property of the sauna is attributed to the following facts:

- Overheating stimulates and speeds up the metabolic processes and inhibits the growth of virus, bacteria.
- All the vital organs and glands are stimulated to increased activity.
- The body's healing forces are aided and assisted, and healing is accelerated.
- The eliminative, detoxifying and cleansing capacity of the skin is increased by the profuse sweating.

NOTE: Although fever is a natural, constructive, beneficial symptom, and fever therapy is one of the most effective means in the arsenal of biological modalities, I must stress the fact that fever therapy should always be supervised by an expert practitioner and undertaken on the advice of a doctor. The patient's heart condition, his ability to perspire and his general vitality should be checked and his reaction during the therapy closely supervised. Also, the length of the overheating therapy should be determined by the doctor.

The above warning is in regard to patients who are ill. There is, of course, no danger for healthy people to take sauna or other steam or hot baths on a regular basis as a preventive, cleansing and health-building measure, as millions of people are doing both here and in Europe.

Reference: How to get well by Paavo Airola, 1974, page 241-242

Strengthening the Body's Natural Defenses

Integrative Medicine will make a difference in cancer care by the late Dr. David Servan-Schreiber, MD, a 20 year cancer survivor and author of Anticancer: A New Way of Life:

"Integrative medicine aims to enhance cancer care by creating a comprehensive, integrative treatment plan that addresses all dimensions of care – physical, psychological-spiritual, and social. It makes use of all appropriate therapeutic approaches, providers, and disciplines to improve quality of life, help to manage symptoms, and achieve the best possible treatment results.

Recent research shows that tumors grow and become malignant not only through genetic anomalies in the cancer cells themselves, but also through factors in the cells' microenvironment. These microenvironmental factors include, but are not limited to, the ability of the cells to form blood vessels to feed the growing tumor (angiogenesis), the propensity for inflammation and stimulating inflammatory pathways, and suppressed cell-mediated immunity. The tumor microenvironment is the terrain that largely determines whether cancerous cells will grow or not. The body possesses a number of natural defenses that can create a barren, inhospitable terrain for cancer growth. These natural defenses are influenced and strengthened by healthy lifestyle choices such as a proper diet, physical activity, stress management, social connection, and limiting exposure to environmental pollutants.

Modern oncology treatment is focused on destroying cancer cells or blocking cancer-related pathways. This is an essential aspect of therapy. However, it is becoming increasingly clear that truly effective cancer care should simultaneously foster a strong anticancer terrain by strengthening the body's natural defenses. Existing initial research that follows the tenets of integrative oncology (making changes in lifestyle and behavior) shows evidence that this approach can, in fact, strengthen natural defenses, modify the terrain of the body, and have an impact on long-term treatment results.

It is time to provide our patients the education and clinical tools necessary to support an anti-cancer lifestyle to help them remain cancer free and to improve clinical outcomes, quality of life, and symptom control for those with cancer and cancer survivors. We need to empower people to become active participants in their own health. We need to show them how to best care for themselves; not only because they will feel better if they get involved, but because it's good science and good medicine." See Strengthening Natural Defenses at http://keystohealing.ca and anticancerbook.com

Source: Anti Cancer: A New Way of Life by Dr. David Servan-Schreiber, MD, PhD, Feb 25, 2010

It is a fact that Chinese medicine has used cannabis (Ma Fen) as a healing herb for millennia according to The Divine Farmer's Materia Medica (Shen Nung Ben Cao Jing). However, Traditional Chinese medicine physicians are dedicated Qigong, herbal and acupuncture practitioners so they have the skills to harness the transformative healing potential of cannabis, and neutralize its mild side-effects. Self-medicating with cannabis without the Chinese medicine knowledge and therapies, and Qigong training can make existing symptoms worse or create other imbalances.

Western research has confirmed that cannabis, Qigong and acupuncture work with the endocannabinoid system of the body, and a specific type of acupuncture can heal pain, anxiety, depression, addiction and deliver that great stoned feeling similar to cannabis. Therefore, medical cannabis can revolutionize the practice of TCM because the body's endocannabinoid system is activated to heal diseases. Additionally, Qigong and acupuncture are definitely needed to balance Qi in the body when cannabis is taken.

References:

1. The Cancer Industry: The Classic Expose on the Cancer Establishment by Ralph W. Moss, 1991; Cancer's Cause, Cancer's Cure by M. Walker, 2012
2. Options: the Alternative Cancer Therapy Book by Richard Walters, 1993
3. What is Cancer? By Dr. Joseph Gold at thepathogenesisofcancer.com, scri.ngen.com, hydrazinesulfate.org
4. Dr. Gold Speaks by Dr. Joseph Gold at medtruth.blogspot.com
5. Tyramine-Rich Foods by Theodore G Tong, Pharm D/C Hansen and Stephen R. Saklad, Pharm.D
6. Alkaline Ionized Water: qigonghealer.com/water.html Ricardo B Serrano
7. Cessiac & Yuccalive: The Cure & Cause of Cancer is Within You at holisticwebs.com/cancer/cancer.html by Ricardo B Serrano, R.Ac.
8. Reishi Mushroom: from Ron Teeguarden's book Radiant Health, the Ancient Wisdom of the Chinese Tonic Herbs
9. Dr. Budwig's Diet by Ricardo B Serrano, R.Ac. qigongmastery.ca
10. You Hold the Keys to Healing by Ricardo B Serrano, R.Ac. keystohealing.ca
11. How to Conquer Death Now: Oneness with Shiva by Ricardo B Serrano, RAc
12. Hydrazine Sulfate at Life Energy Distributor lifepharma.com
13. Cancer and Hydrazine Sulfate from http://www.rifevidoes.com
14. Encyclopedia and Dictionary of Medicine and Nursing, by Miller & Keane
15. Gluconeogenesis Chart by C. Ophandt, 2003.
16. Fats and Oils by Udo Erasmus, 1986.
17. Pranic Healing by Grand Master Choa Kok Sui, 1990.
18. Chinese Medical Qigong Therapy with Sheng Zhen Wuji Yuan Gong
19. Testimonial on Pan Gu Shen Gong by Tan Caixia
20. Healing Power of Rainforest Herbs by Leslie Taylor, ND 2004, rain-tree.com
21. Health Sciences Institute (HSI) Newsletter, hsionline.com
22. Does Guyabano Cure Cancer? by Ricardo B Serrano, R.Ac. keystohealing.ca
23. Dr. Beljanski's herbals for cancer at beljanski.com and natural-source.com
24. Anti Cancer: A New Way of Life by Dr. David Servan-Schreiber, 2008.
25. The Coconut Oil Miracle and Coco Ketogenic Diet by Dr. Bruce Fife, 2014.
26. Rick Simpson Oil, Nature's Cure for Cancer, 2015
27. Marijuana Medicine by Christian Ratsch, 2001
28. Marijuana Medical Handbook by Dale Gieringer, PhD, 2008
29. Cannabis Pharmacy by Michael Backes, 2014
30. Stoned A Doctor's Case for Medical Marijuana by Dave Casarett, MD, 2015

*With thanks and acknowledgements to all the above authors and creators.

GLOSSARY

Adenosine: a nucleotide containing adenine, a pentose sugar and phosphoric acid, which functions as a coenzyme in the metabolic functions of the cell. Adenosine plays a role in the activation of fatty acids and amino acids, and in "energy trapping" in the metabolism of carbohydrates. Nucleosides such as adenosine are believed to be intermediates in the synthesis or degradation of nucleic acids.

   a. diphosphate, a compound containing two phosphoric acids, formed by hydrolysis of adenosine triphosphate, with release of one high-energy bond; abbreviated ADP
      a. monophosphate, adenosine containing only one phosphoric acid; abbreviated ADP
         a. triphosphate (ATP), compound containing three phosphoric acids, with one low- and two high-energy bonds; abbreviated ATP

Angiogenesis: growth of new blood vessels in tumors. See *Taheebo, hemp oil* and *Curcumin*

Annonaceous Acetogenins: found only in the plant family *Annonaceae* (**Guyabano**) Chemically, they are derivatives of long-chain fatty acids. Biologically, the primary site of action of the *acetogenins* is complex I of the electron transport in mitochondria. The *acetogenins* are also inhibitors of the NADH (Nicotinamide adenine dinucleotide) oxidase which is prevalent in the plasma membranes of cancer cells. Both modes of action deplete ATP and induce program cell death. Cancer cells are better targets for the *acetogenins* than normal cells because they have elevated levels of NADH oxidase accompanied by higher ATP demand. "Guyabano's (Graviola) leaves and fruit grown in the Philippines is a miracle cancer cure according to the Filipinos I have interviewed." – Ricardo B Serrano

Cachexia: a state of malnutrition, emaciation and debility, usually in the course of a chronic illness like cancer.

Cancer: any malignant tumor. Adj., cancerous. Cancer is a neoplastic disease in which there is new growth of abnormal cells. Normally the cells that compose body tissues grow in response to a normal stimulus. Worn-out body cells are regularly replaced by new cell growth which stops when the cells are replaced; new cells form to repair tissue damage and stop forming when healing is complete. Why they stop forming is unknown, but clearly the body in its normal processes regulates cell growth. In cancer, cell growth is unregulated. The cells continue to reproduce until they form a mass of tissue known as tumor. Not all tumors are malignant; those which are non-cancerous are referred to as benign tumors. **Benign tumors** vary in size, and may grow so large that they obstruct organs or cause ulceration and bleeding. They are encapsulated, do not metastasize and usually can be removed by surgery without difficulty.

Malignant tumors grow in a disorganized fashion, interrupting body functions and robbing normal cells of their food and blood supply. The malignant cells may spread to other parts of the body by (1) direct extension into adjacent tissue, (2) permeation along lymphatic vessels (3) traveling in the lymph stream to the lymph nodes, (4) entering the blood circulation and (5) invasion of body cavity by diffusion.

Classification. Cancers are divided into two large groups; Sarcomas and Carcinomas. Sarcomas are of mesenchymal origin and affect such tissues as the bones and muscles. They tend to grow rapidly and to be very destructive. The carcinomas are of epithelial origin and make up the great majority of the glandular cancers and cancers of the breast, stomach, uterus, skin and tongue.

Precancers. Some potentially dangerous cancers appear first in the form of harmless changes in the body's tissues. Their danger lies in the fact that they have a tendency to become malignant. Hence they are known as precancers.

Among these are sores that appear as thickened white patches (leukoplakia) in the mouth and in the vulva, some moles and any chronically irritated area on the skin or the mucous membranes of the mouth and tongue. Polyps also are possible precancers as are some forms of lymphomas.

Hodgkin's Disease. This disease is generally considered a form of cancer. It usually afflicts young people, causing a progressive enlargement of the lymph nodes, in most cases starting in the neck, groin or armpit. Treatment maybe surgery, radiotherapy, use of certain chemicals or a combination of these.

Leukemias. In these diseases, abnormal leukocytes are produced in enormous quantities. The leukemias respond to much the same treatment as cancer and are commonly considered cancers.

Symptoms of Cancer. There are seven early warning signs of cancer. These signs do not necessarily signify cancer, but should they occur, a physician should be consulted and an examination is advisable, Other symptoms depend on location and type of malignancy present.

Early Danger Signs of Cancer

1. Any lump or thickening, especially in the breast, lip or tongue.
2. Any irregular or unexplained bleeding. Blood in the urine or bowel movements. Blood or bloody discharge from the nipple of anybody opening. Unexplained vaginal bleeding or discharge, or any bleeding after the menopause.
3. A sore that does not heal, particularly around the mouth, tongue or lips, or anywhere on the skin.
4. Noticeable changes in the color or size of a wart, mole or birthmark.
5. Loss of appetite or continual indigestion.
6. Persistent hoarseness, cough or difficulty in swallowing.
7. Persistent change in normal elimination (bowel habits). **Special Note**: Pain is not usually an early warning sign of cancer.

Stomach cancer: continued lack of appetite; persistent indigestion; pain after eating; loss of weight; vomiting; anemia.

Cancer of the rectum: changes in bowel habits, such as periods of constipation followed by episodes of diarrhea; abnormal cramps and a sensation of incomplete elimination or a feeling that there is a mass in the rectum; rectal pain and bleeding.

Cancer of the uterus; increased or irregular vaginal discharges; return of vaginal bleeding after the menopause; bleeding between menstrual periods or after coitus.

Cancer of the breast: painless lumps in the breast; bleeding or discharging from the nipple. Many kinds of lumps in the breast are innocent, but since this form of cancer is now the leading cause of death from cancer among women, any breast module or tumor should be examined by a physician.

Skin cancer: sores and ulcers that do not heal; sudden changes in color, size and texture in moles, warts, scars and birthmarks.

Lung cancer: a persistent cough that lasts beyond 2 weeks; wheezing or other noises in the chest; coughing up blood or bloody sputum; shortness of breath not caused by obvious exertion, such as climbing stairs or running; chest ache or pain.

Cancer of the mouth, tongue and lips: any sore that does not heal in 2 weeks; any white patch taking the place of the normal pink color of the tongue or inside of the mouth; hoarseness lasting more than 2 weeks. **Cancer of the larynx**: persistent hoarseness.

Kidney, bladder and prostate cancers: bloody urine or reddish or pink urine; difficulty in starting urination; increasing frequency of urination during the night,

Brain tumors and cancers: headaches; changes in vision; dizziness; nausea and vomiting; paralysis.

Diagnosis: The detection of cancer can be accomplished by a number of tests and examinations. By palpation, a tumor can be felt as a lamp or nodule below the surface of the skin or mucous membrane. By visualization of the hollow organs with instruments such as the cytoscope, proctoscope, or bronchoscope, abnormal growths of cells can be seen. Laboratory examination of the cells removed by biopsy can determine whether a tumor is malignant or benign. This test is considered the more accurate and dependable aid to diagnosis of cancer.

The *papanicolaou smear test* is used for diagnosing early cancers of the uterine cervix, mouth, bronchi, stomach and other organs lined with mucous membrane. In this technique washings or scrapings from the mucous membrane are removed by the physician, placed on a glass slide and sent to a laboratory for cytologic examination. Radiologic studies, using x-ray films and fluoroscopy, can reveal tumors which may not be detected by other means. In addition to gastrointestinal studies, chest x-rays and pyelography, radiologic studies for cancer include angiography and mammograohy. Radioisotopes and photoscanners may be used to locate tumors of the brain, pancreas, thyroid, liver and kidney. In this method the radioactive compound is introduced into the body orally or by injection. The compound travels through the body and localizes in a specific organ. Special instruments are used to trace and "photograoh" the abnormal collection of radioisotopes, thereby pinpointing the location of the tumor.

There is at present no general chemical test of the blood by which malignant growths can be distinguished from benign. The blood can be tested chemically for cancer of the prostate and for a rare malignancy of the bone marrow called multiple myeloma. A blood count can also help in the diagnosis of leukemias.

Treatment. The present methods of treating cancer are surgery, radiation and chemotherapy. Surgical removal of the tumor is aimed at removal of all cancerous tissue and is most frequently successful if undertaken when the growth is still small and localized. The goal of radiotherapy is also the complete destruction of all malignant tissue. Radiation damages tissue, particularly tissue that is growing. Since malignant tissue grows rapidly, it is more readily destroyed than normal body tissue.

The type of radiation to be used is determined by the radiologist, depending upon the nature and location of the cancerous growth. He may use x-rays or gamma rays. Gamma rays are similar in nature to x-rays, but they are usually more powerful and penetrating. If the cancer is accessible, this deep radiation therapy may not be necessary. In some cases, radiation sources in the form of radium or radioisotopes can be embedded directly in the cancer and removed when the desired dose has been delivered.

Of the chemicals and drugs used in treating cancer, the most widely used are compounds known as the nitrogen mustards. These are composed of various combinations of carbon, hydrogen, chlorine and nitrogen, and are similar in some respects to the poisonous mustard gas used in World War 1. Their effect is to shrink and otherwise retard the growth of the cancer. These and other compounds such as folic acid antagonists, corticosteroids, purine analogues, alkaloids and alkylating agents have been found particularly valuable in treating leukemias and Hodgkin's disease, and have been helpful in some cases of cancer of the ovaries and advanced lung cancer.

Researchers are constantly testing other substances, a number of which are showing promise. Radioactive iodine, mixed in water and given orally, has been used to help treat some rare cancers of the thyroid gland. An antibiotic, actinomycin D, used together with surgery and radiation, has been of value in children treated for a kidney cancer known as Wilms' tumor.

Also of use in treating cancer are various hormones. Female hormones have been found effective in some cases of cancer of the prostate, and male hormones are frequently helpful in treating cancer of the breast.

Deoxyribonucleic acid DNA: a nucleic acid that is a large complex molecule composed of phosphoric acid, a pentose (deoxyribose) and a mixture of purines and pyrimidines. DNA is the basic substance of GENES and carries the code of genetic information controlling development of the organism. DNA is a double molecule, capable of reproducing itself and also of producing ribonucleic acid (RNA), which in turn produces proteins. Since protein is the essential material of protoplasm, the importance of DNA in the vitality of the cell is obvious. The ability of DNA to reproduce itself explains how genes can reproduce again and again without changing their individual characteristics. See **beljanski.com**

Enzyme: a substance, usually protein in nature, that initiates and accelerates a chemical reaction.

Gluconeogenesis: the formation of sugar by the liver from noncarbohydrate molecules such as lactic acid.

Glucose: a simple sugar, called also dextrose; the principal monosaccharide in human blood and body fluids.

Glycolysis: the breaking down of sugars into simpler compounds. Adj. glycolytic

Hydrazine sulfate: the salt of hydrazine and sulfuric acid. Known by the trade name Sehydrin, it is a chemical compound that has been used as an alternative medical treatment for the loss of appetite (anorexia) and weight loss (cachexia) which is often associated with cancer.

Lactic acid: a compound formed in the body in anaerobic metabolism of carbohydrate, and also produced by bacterial action on milk.

Monoamine oxidase is found in the gastrointestinal tract and inactivates tyramine; when drugs prevent the catabolism of exogenous tyramine, this amino acid is absorbed and displaces norepinephrine from sympathetic nerve ending and epinephrine from the adrenal glands.

Monoamine oxidase inhibitors (MAOIs) are chemicals which inhibit the activity of the monoamine oxidase enzyme family.

Oxidation: the act of oxidizing or state of being oxidized. Adj., oxidative. Chemically it consists in the increase of positive charges on an atom or the loss of negative charges. Univalent oxidation indicates loss of one electron; divalent oxidation, the loss of two electrons. The opposite reaction to oxidation is reduction. **Oxidize**: to cause to combine with oxygen.

Tumor: 1. Swelling, one of the cardinal signs of inflammation. 2. A swelling or enlargement due to pathologic overgrowth of tissue. Adj. tumorous. Tumors are called also neoplasms, which means that they are composed of new and actively growing tissue. Their growth is faster than that of normal tissue, continuing after cessation of the stimuli that evoked the growth, and serving no useful physiologic purpose.

Tumors are classified in a number of ways, one of the simplest being according to their origin and whether they are malignant or benign. Tumors of mesenchymal origin include fibroelastic tumors and those of bone, fat, blood vessels and lymphoid tissue. They maybe benign or malignant (sarcoma). Tumors of epithelial origin maybe benign or malignant (sarcoma); they are found in glandular tissue or such organs as the breast, stomach, uterus or skin. Mixed tumors contain different types of cells derived from the same primary germ layer, and tetratomas contain cells derived from more than one germ layer; both kinds may

Benign tumors. Benign tumors do not endanger life unless they interfere with normal functions of other organs or affect a vital organ. They grow slowly, pushing aside normal tissue but not invading it. They are usually encapsulated, well demarcated growths. They are not metastatic; that is, they do not form secondary tumors in other organs. Benign tumors usually respond favorably to surgical treatment and some form of radiotherapy.

Malignant tumors. These tumors are composed of embryonic. Primitive or poorly differentiated cells. They grow in a disorganized manner and so rapidly that nutrition of the cells becomes a problem. For this reason necrosis and ulceration are characteristic of malignant tumors. They are also invading surrounding tissues and are metastatic, initiating the growth of similar tumors in distant organs.

Senescence: the process of growing old.

Telomere: an extremity of a chromosome, which has specific properties, one of which is failure to fuse with other fragments of chromosomes after a chromosome has been broken.

Tyramine: a decarboxylation product of tyrosine with a similar (but weaker) action to that of epinephrine and norepinephrine, and capable of releasing stored norepinephrine.

Tyrosine: a naturally occurring amino acid produced in the body in the metabolism of phenylalanine to melanin, epinephrine and thyroxine.

Source: Encyclopedia and Dictionary of Medicine and Nursing, by Miller & Keane, 1972, Fats and Oils by Udo Erasmus, 1986, and Health Sciences Institute (HSI).

Treating depression, chronic pain and anxiety disorders with medical cannabis and photobiomodulation

To experience occasional sadness and anxiety are a normal part of life.

Some people, however, due to stress, cancer, chronic pain, addiction or trauma experience sadness or anxiety in such a manner that it starts disturbing their job performance, school work and even relationships. They have what is called major depression or anxiety disorder.

- The symptoms of major depression include lingering sadness or irritability, loss of motivation and zest for living, a pessimistic or worrisome attitude, changes in sleep pattern, changes in appetite and energy level, lower self-worth, poor concentration, forgetfulness, and thoughts of death or suicide.
- Anxiety disorders, on the other hand, manifest in palpitations, breathing difficulties, cold sweat, dizziness or light-headedness, body weakness, tremors, digestive system problems, a sense of panic or uneasiness, fears of going crazy, losing control, and being seriously ill.

The treatment package for major depression, cancer, chronic pain, addiction and anxiety disorders includes herbal medication, spiritual healing, stress management techniques, nutritional supplementation, acupuncture, Qigong, and lifestyle changes. On herbal medication (medical cannabis) alone, significant improvement is usually seen in two to three weeks of taking the right herbal medication at the right dose. The right herbal medication is one that is natural, effective, non-habit forming, and without side-effects. Cannabis is also used as an aid to psychotherapy and an agent to ease withdrawal from alcohol and opiates. See **Holistic Biochemistry of Cannabinoids, p. 20**

Photobiomodulation by Vielight Neuro Gamma is a non-drug approach that not only works to heal depression but also works for cancer-related anxiety, insomnia, fatigue, pain, and cognitive impairment. See Photobiomodulation, pages 46, 103, 111, 135

It Works (Abstract) How Cannabinoids Kill Cancer Cells by Biochemist Dennis Hill, prostate cancer survivor

This brief survey touches lightly on a few essential concepts. Mostly I would like to leave you with an appreciation that nature has designed the perfect medicine that fits exactly with our own immune system of receptors and signaling metabolites to provide rapid and complete immune response for systemic integrity and metabolic homeostasis. - Dennis Hill

"My opinion is that oral cannabis extract with equal parts THC and CBD is the ideal cancer killer without the mental effects. The cannabinoids work in concert to kill cancer; this is known as the entourage effect; THC disrupts the cancer cell mitochondria, and CBD disrupts the cell's endoplasmic reticulum, bringing certain cell death." – Biochemist Dennis Hill

There is a plentiful supply of research articles and personal testaments that show the efficacy of cannabis effecting cancer remission. However, only a few point to the mechanism by which the cancer cells die. To understand this better we need to know what metabolic processes provide life to the cells.

There are two structures in most cells that sustains life; one is the mitochondria, and the other is the endoplasmic reticulum. The mitochondria primarily produces adenosine triphosphate (ATP) that provides the necessary energy. The endoplasmic reticulum (ER) is a loosely bound envelope around the cell nucleus that synthesizes metabolites and proteins directed by the nuclear DNA that nourish and sustain the cell.

Let us look first at tetrahydrocannabinol (THC) and observe that THC is a natural fit for the CB1 cannabinoid receptor on the cancer cell surface. When THC hits the receptor, the cell generates ceramide that disrupts the mitochondria, closing off energy for the cell.

Disruption of the mitochondria releases cytochrome c and reactive oxygen species into the cytosol, hastening cell death. It is notable that this process is specific to cancer cells. Healthy cells have no reaction to THC at the CB1 receptor. The increase in ceramide also disrupts calcium metabolism in the mitochondria, completing the demise to cell death.

The other cannabinoid we know is effective in killing cancer cells is cannabidiol (CBD). The primary job of CBD in the cancer cell is to disrupt the endoplasmic reticulum through wrecking of the calcium metabolism, pushing calcium into the cytosol. This always results in cell death. Another pathway for CBD to effect cancer cell death is the Caspase Cascade, which breaks down proteins and peptides in the cell. When this happens the cell cannot survive. Again, these processes are specific to cancer cells, no normal cells are affected.

References: How Medical Cannabis Works, page 19; Holistic Biochemistry of Cannabinoids, page 20; Cancer and Cannabis Medicines, page 26; Endocannabinoid Deficiency, page 112; Final Notes on Rick Simpson cannabis hemp oil, page 134

Reference:

1. The Journal of Neuroscience, February 18, 2009 • 29(7):2053–2063 • 2053
   Cannabidiol Targets Mitochondria to Regulate Intracellular Calcium Levels.
   Duncan Ryan, Alison J. Drysdale, Carlos Lafourcade, Roger G. Pertwee, and Bettina Platt.
   School of Medical Sciences, University of Aberdeen, Foresterhill, Aberdeen AB25 2ZD, United Kingdom.
2. Mol Cancer Ther July 2011 10; 1161
   Cannabidiol Induces Programmed Cell Death in Breast Cancer Cells by Coordinating the Cross-talk between Apoptosis and Autophagy
   Ashutosh Shrivastava, Paula M. Kuzontkoski, Jerome E. Groopman, and Anil Prasad.
   Division of Experimental Medicine, Beth Israel Deaconess Medical Center, Harvard Medical School, Boston, Massachusetts.

Anti-Cancer Action (excerpts from AntiCancer: A New Way of Life by Dr. Servan-Schreiber)

Common promoters of cancer are:

1. Cigarette smoke and more than one alcoholic beverage (red wine) per day. Vaccination is also a factor to consider as a causative factor in certain forms of cancer.
2. Refined sugar and white flour (corn syrup, sodas, cakes, doughnuts, etc)
3. Omega-6 fatty acids and trans-fats (corn, soybean, sunflower and safflower oils, hydrogenated and partially hydrogenated vegetable oils
4. A variety of chemical agents present in some foods and household products (parabens, phthalates, PVCs, pesticides and herbicides)
5. Complete lack of physical activity
6. Responses to stress that lead to feelings of helplessness and persistent despair rather than a sense that one can help oneself or count on the support of others

Factors that slow down the growth of cancer are:

1. Several phytochemicals contained in some fruits and some vegetables, some herbs and spices(turmeric, mint, thyme, rosemary, garlic, guyabano)
2. Omega-3 fatty acids (fatty fish, canola and flaxseed oil, flaxseeds, walnuts, some green vegetables), and Virgin Coconut Oil rich in Medium Chain Fatty Acid (MCFA)
3. Physical activity (at least 30 minutes of walking six times a week)
4. The ability to manage stress so as to avoid helplessness (emotional management through meditation or yoga or good psychotherapy) or benefiting from the support of intimate relationships, or both.
5. **Diet:** Eat grass-fed organic animal products: meat, milk, cheese, yogurt, omega-3 eggs

Balance your diet, exercise, meditate, and free yourself of your feelings of powerlessness

1. Reduce your intake of sugar, white flour or rice, products containing omega-6s – sunflower oil, corn oil, soybean oil, safflower oil, margarine, hydrogenated (trans) fat, nonorganic animal fat (meat, eggs, dairy products)
2. Increase your omega-3 intake (found in fish, grass- or flaxseed-fed animal products, flaxseed and oil) and Virgin Coconut Oil rich in Medium Chain Triglycerides (MCT)
3. Increase your intake of anticancer products (turmeric, green tea, aratiles, soy, specific anticancer vegetables and fruits) See Coconut Ketogenic Diet, page 121
4. **Filter tap water**: use carbon filter or an inverse osmosis filter or drink mineral water or spring water (alkaline ionized water is much better, in my opinion)
5. **Activity:** Spend 20 to 30 minutes engaged in physical activity per day; Expose yourself to sunlight for 20 minutes each day (creates vitamin D)
6. **Meditation:** Practice a method of relaxation and self-centering (such as yoga, cardiac coherence, Qigong, tai chi, etc). It also replenishes negative ions the body needs for healing.
7. **Free yourself of your feelings of powerlessness:** Resolve past traumas; learn to accept your emotions, including fear, sadness, despair, and anger; find someone with whom you can share your emotions. Knowing that genetics are only a minor contribution to cancer helps us realize how much is in our power to help our body be a stronger partner in nourishing life and resisting cancer.

FINAL NOTES: From an Oriental integrative medical perspective, cancer is a matter of the body's terrain, the tumor microenvironment, and therefore a lifestyle disease.

Everyone has cancer cells in our bodies but not everyone will develop cancer. Why is this? What do we do in the west to "treat the terrain"? This is because cancer is caused by a cancer terrain with the body's weakened natural defenses or immune system brought on with a cancer promoter lifestyle - smoking, drinking, eating high sugar and saturated fat diet, sedentary (non-exercise) habits, unmanaged stress, and social isolation - and can be cured naturally with an anti-cancer lifestyle that fosters an anti-cancer terrain by strengthening the body's natural defenses. Environmental factors such as pollution, chemicals in our food supply and home, and side-effects of prescription and street drugs also contribute to the rising epidemic of cancer, however, without making lifestyle and behavioral changes within ourselves, cancer can't be prevented and survival of cancer survivors will be short-lived.

Recent research shows that tumors grow and become malignant not only through genetic anomalies in the cancer cells themselves, but also through factors in the cells' microenvironment. These microenvironmental factors include, but are not limited to, the ability of the cells to form blood vessels to feed the growing tumor (angiogenesis), the propensity for inflammation and stimulating inflammatory pathways, and suppressed cell-mediated immunity. The tumor microenvironment is the terrain that largely determines whether cancerous cells will grow or not. The body possesses a number of natural defenses that can create a barren, inhospitable terrain for cancer growth. These natural defenses are influenced and strengthened by healthy lifestyle choices such as a proper diet, physical activity, stress management, social connection, and limiting exposure to environmental pollutants.

Finally, cannabis hemp oil popularized by Rick Simpson at his website http://phoenixtears.ca should be tried by any cancer sufferer before using invasive medical therapies such as chemotherapy, surgery and radiation. He has assisted thousands of cancer patients through his instructions in how to make cannabis hemp oil in his website. Hemp oil is not only excellent for curing cancer but also other chronic diseases such as diabetes, high blood pressure, arthritis, asthma, depression, sleeping problems, MS, Parkinson's, inflammation and drug and alcohol addictions. Hemp oil can be mixed with coconut oil for best results.

There are a significant amount of studies that show THC and CBD compounds found within cannabis, known as cannabinoids, have anti-cancer properties. The United States' National Institute of Health stated that: "Cannabinoids may cause antitumor effects by various mechanisms, including induction of cell death, inhibition of cell growth, and inhibition of tumor angiogenesis invasion and metastasis." Antiangiogenesis prevents the formation of new blood vessels needed by tumor to grow.

This book and the other six books in *You Hold the Keys to Healing,* based from my research and experience of my clients and patients as a long time integrative Chinese medical practitioner, will assist your nutrition and meditation and Qigong practices, and free yourself of your feelings of powerlessness or hopelessness fostering a strong anticancer terrain by strengthening the body's natural defenses. Following an anti-cancer lifestyle will not only prevent and treat cancer but prevent and treat other degenerative diseases as well.

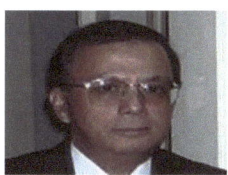

Master Pranic Healer Ricardo B Serrano, R.Ac, a registered acupuncturist, integrates pranic healing with Enlightenment Qigong forms, acupuncture, herbs and acupressure. He is a certified Qigong teacher trained by Pan Gu Shen Gong Master Ou Wen Wei, Sheng Zhen Gong Master Li Junfeng, Qi Dao Master Lama Tantrapa, Primordial Wuji Qigong Master Michael Winn, Zhan Zhuang Qigong Master Richard Mooney, Pranic Healing Grand Master Choa Kok Sui, Master Nona Castro and Mang Mike Nator. He is also a certified Merkabah teacher trained by Merkabah Master Alton Kamadon and Sri Vidya teacher Raja Choudhury. He is a Master Herbalist from Dominion Herbal College and Certified Cannabis Specialist from Cannabis Hemp Academy.

His seven books Return to Oneness with Shiva, Oneness with Shiva, Return to Oneness with the Tao, Return to Oneness with Spirit, Meditation and Qigong Mastery, and Keys to Healing and Self-Mastery, and The Cure & Cause of Cancer comprise altogether his Master Pranic Healer thesis for the Integral Studies of Inner Sciences.

His blogsites are: freedomhealthrecovery.com/blog, keystohealing.ca, and innerway.ca His websites are: holisticwebs.com, freedomhealthrecovery.com, qigonghealer.com, qiwithoutborders.org, and qigongmastery.ca You can contact Acharya Ricardo B Serrano through his websites for Shaktipat, meditation, and Qigong workshops and for his functional medicine Oriental medical therapies – acupuncture, acupressure, herbal consultations and Qi-healing (pranic healing) with Qigong - for drug dependency, cancer and degenerative disease conditions.

Ricardo has been to his native country, Philippines, for four months (December till March, 2013) to research material for his book "The Cure & Cause of Cancer" and he has found powerful herbs used by Filipinos such as aratiles, Pau d' Arco (Taheebo), Turmeric, an angiogenesis inhibitor, and Guyabano (Graviola) as their main herbs used for alternative cancer therapy. These three herbs together with Cessiac and Chaparral mentioned in the book should not be taken with MAO inhibitor medications and other medications. Risk information for each of these herbs is included in the book for your safety as a prevention for contraindications with MAO inhibitor medication and other synthetic medications, and also tyramine-rich foods.

Guyabano's (Graviola) leaves and fruit grown in the Philippines is a miracle cancer cure according to the Filipinos he has interviewed. The main reason is that graviola is an effective cancer fighter stems from a research (published in 2008) conducted at the Purdue University's School of Pharmacy and Pharmaceutical Sciences on the unique substances known as **annonaceous acetogenins** that have been extracted from the graviola tree.

Kerson Fruit or Muntingia calabura (aratiles) is a fast growing tree that has a cherry like fruit with multiple health benefits: Such as antibacterial, lowering blood sugar, preventing cancer, promoting cardiovascular health, lowering blood pressure, and blocking pain (gout, headaches) … just to name a few. According to research, the leaves of the Kerson tree demonstrates great anti-cancer abilities and may be utilized more widely in the future for cancer cure – additional studies required.

Intranasal light therapy together with Guo Lin Qigong, and an electromagnetic healing technology device invented in the Philippines can rebuild the body's Qi field by supplying negative ions and nitric oxide needed to heal cancer and other chronic diseases.

CoQ10 is key to our heart health. It's crucial to protecting your mitochondria. It is key to delaying or preventing mitochondrial depletion. Ubiquinol supplementation with Magnesium is best integrated with intranasal light therapy for healing diseases.

The Vielight intranasal light therapy (ILT) is an indispensable therapy as maintenance medicine that supply the healing near infrared light energy nasally to normalize blood pressure, blood sugar, blood cholesterol, hormonal levels; reduce aches and pain, improve mood and sleep, and adds vital energy to physical performance and higher meditation practices**.** ILT also penetrates deep enough into the nasal cavity to gently stimulate a homeostatic (balancing effect) on the midbrain including the hypothalamus. The hypothalamus is a critical part of your brain that communicates with your pituitary gland to exert influence over a variety of hormone functions.

ILT is an alternative non-invasive therapy to the IV laser therapy invented in Russia that is practiced by irradiating the blood with laser beam intravenously. The cellular mechanisms and health benefits of IV laser therapy is similar to the cellular mechanisms and health benefits derived from ILT.

According to scientific research, Intranasal light therapy with 633 nm, stimulates the mitochondria to produce more ATP, and triggers the release of nitric oxide (NO), a powerful cell signaler and activator. NO sends "blood flow signals" that relax arterial walls, dilate the blood vessels, and improve the flow of blood and oxygen everywhere in your body, boosting its ability to heal obesity, heart disease, cancer, Alzheimer's, stroke, arthritis, high blood pressure, and of course diabetes.

It is also used to reduce anxiety and pain, improve mood and performance, and enter higher meditative states of consciousness by stimulating Qi in the acupuncture meridians improving the Qi flow in the Wei Qi field restoring homeostasis systemically. Light energy (Qi) is absorbed by the blood vessels in the nasal cavity via intranasal light therapy. According to Chinese medicine, blood provides a carrier for the movement of Qi and nourishes it. Sufficient blood and good blood circulation is essential to maintaining strong Qi for true healing and enlightenment Light is truly the medicine of the future.

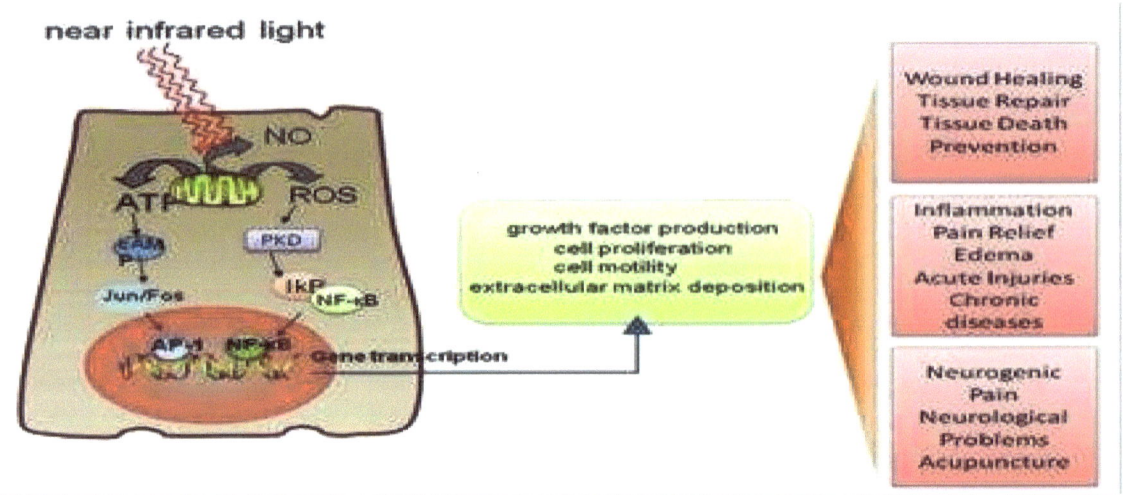

www.ingramcontent.com/pod-product-compliance
Lightning Source LLC
Chambersburg PA
CBHW041549220426
43666CB00002B/19